15,048/50

EPONYMISTS IN MEDICINE

Alzheimer and the Dementias

Editors

G. E. Berrios and H. L. Freeman

Editor-in-Chief: Hugh L'Etang

Royal Society of Medicine Services Limited

Royal Society of Medicine Services Limited
1 Wimpole Street London W1M 8AE
7 East 60th Street New York NY 10022

British Library Cataloguing in Publication Data

Alzheimer and the dementias.—(Eponymists in
  medicine, ISSN 0955-8640)
  I. Berrios, G. E. (German Elias) II. Freeman, Hugh
  III. Series
  616.8092

  ISBN 1-85315-157-2

Design by Mehmet Hussein/Medilink Design

Phototypeset by Dobbie Typesetting Limited, Tavistock, Devon

Printed in Great Britain by Henry Ling Ltd, at the Dorset Press, Dorchester

Contents

Illustrations

Notable Events in Alzheimer's Lifetime

	Alzheimer	World of Science	World Events
1864	Born on 14th June	Death of Marcé	Bismarck attacks Denmark
1865			End of American Civil War; Assassination of Lincoln
1866		Birth of Adolf Meyer	
1869			Opening of Suez Canal & USA Transcontinental railroad
1870		Birth of Robert Gaupp	Franco-Prussian War & Rocke-feller S Oil Co.
1874		Kahlbaum's book on catatonia	Telephone patented by Bell
1880			
1883	Finished school	Birth of K Jaspers	Death of Richard Wagner
1884	Starts University at Würzburg	Word 'neuron' used	
1888	Starts work in Frankfurt		Death of Mathew Arnold
1890		Kraepelin to Heidelberg	Fall of Bismarck
1894	Marriage		Death of Oliver W Holmes
1893		Death of Charcot	
1895		Röntgen discovers X-Ray	
1898	Paper on senile dementia		Spanish-American War
1899		Death of Kahlbaum	Boer War Starts
1900		Freud's 'Inter-pretation of Dreams'	
1901	Wife dies		Death of Queen Victoria
1903	Heidelberg & Munich	Death of Herbert Spencer	Flight by Wright Brothers

	Alzheimer	World of Science	World Events
1904	Lecturer in Munich	Death of Gilles de la Tourette	Roosevelt speech on 'the incapacity of Philippino people to govern themselves'
1905		Death of Wernicke	Einstein's theory of relativity
1906		Gaupp leaves for Tübingen	
1907	Report of first case of Alzheimer's disease		Picasso and Braque exhibit in Paris
1911	Long paper on the disease	Death of H Jackson	Chinese revolution
1912	Starts work in Breslau		Loss of the Titanic
1914		Death of EA Spitzka	First World War starts
1915	Dies on 19th December	Death of Gowers, Clouston, and Bastian	New USA Immigrants Bill

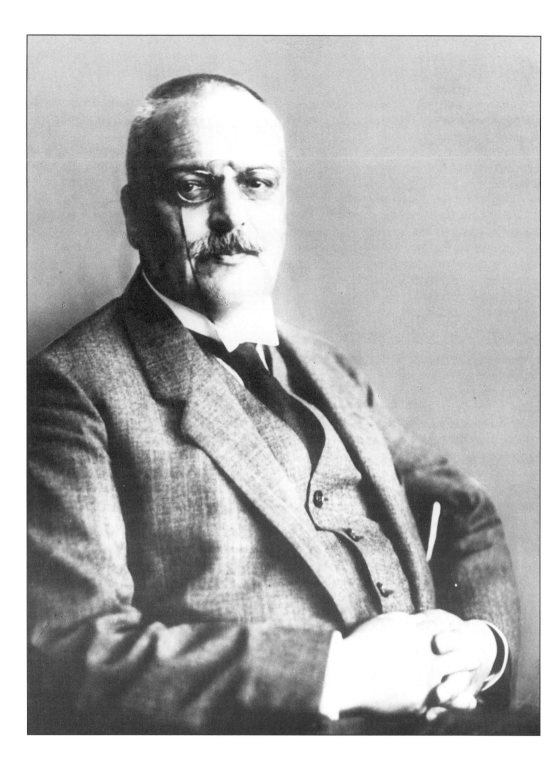

Alois Alzheimer, 1864–1915

Chapter 1

Introduction

G. E. Berrios and H. L. Freeman

Two metaphors are common in the historical study of medicine. In one, the clinician is pictured as cataloguing species in an exotic garden; in the other, as a sculptor carving shapes out of formless matter—creating clinical forms. Yet the one approach needs to explain why the 'naturalist' happens to be there in the first place, and why was he looking at these particular cases, while the other requires an understanding of the contemporary scientific and social constraints on the sculptor's 'inner vision'.

To the consumers of disease, though, it matters little which allegory has been chosen: patients wear their illnesses in the most personal of ways. For their part, clinicians mostly accept the textbook definitions of their time, which are seen as reflecting some 'given' entity—a disease concept which then seems immutable. Yet how far are we ever justified in departing from the criteria originally laid down by the person who first described a particular malady[1]? McMenemey's answer was that differences in neuropathology might be allowed if the case histories remained typical, while symptomatic or clinical differences might be, if the neuropathology was still as first described. So far as Alzheimer's disease is concerned, both types of change have in fact taken place to some extent, since the time of its first description.

Since the 'original' cases of Alzheimer's disease bear only a limited resemblance to those defined by today's criteria, one way out of this impasse has been to assume that the discoverer did not get it quite right. In other words, that Alzheimer and his contemporaries were partially 'wrong' in insisting on the presence of hallucinations and delusions, or in not excluding major arteriosclerotic changes from their concept of the disorder. Perhaps as a consequence of these problems, there has been a recent shift towards the 'creational' approach, which assumes that there is no such a thing as the *final* description of a disease: its clinical boundaries, symptom-content, and even anatomical description are no more than temporary scripts, taken from the ongoing medical discourse[2]. From this point of view, the definition of a disease depends not only on the actual capacities of contemporary science, but also on backroom decisions, taken by her mandarins.

So, in trying to understand why Alzheimer's disease is not called, e.g. Fischer's, Fuller's, or Perusini's disease, the clinician needs to know how nosological categories are derived. These result in fact from the interaction between a descriptive language on the one hand and a biological process (bodily changes which emit signals, in the shape of symptoms and signs) on the other. But the language of description reflects the beliefs of its users, and so the creation of disease is also a social phenomenon. This explains why the 'behavioural' or 'psychiatric' symptoms of Alzheimer's disease were ignored: by the time of the First World War, a purely 'cognitive' view of dementia had been accepted[3]. Recent interest in this issue[4], then, reflects less a change in the presentation of the disease than in the way it is observed by clinicians.

At the end of the nineteenth century, the term 'dementia' was used to name any state of psychological dilapidation associated with chronic brain disease[5,6]. Since deficit states from the functional psychoses were included under this term, irreversibility was not then considered a requirement of dementia[7,8], though efforts had been made ever since the 1820s to relate the two[9]. When states of dementia occurred in the elderly, they were called 'senile dementia'; even as late as 1900, 'dementia' did not necessarily evoke an association with old age, as it mostly does now. This is why neither Morel in the 1860s nor Kraepelin 40 years later had any difficulty using the term—as in 'dementia praecox'—to refer to states of psychological deterioration in young people[10].

Around 1900, a condition of this kind was believed to result from a primary disorder in cognitive function, and was defined almost entirely in terms of the decline of memory[11-14]. Some traditionalists, though, still adhered to the older view that the psychosocial incompetence was not necessarily related to memory impairment: Courbon stated that in dementia, memory 'is in fact much less impaired than it seems' (p300), and believed that the central problem was one of chronic confusion[15]. This explains why, even then, little difficulty was caused by the view that either temporary or permanent remissions might occur in the course of a dementing disease.

The view that dementia was both a clinical and a neuropathological category had been proposed by Bayle as early as 1822[16], though no clear idea existed as to what type of lesions were involved, or whether they all affected the same area of the brain. From the 1860s, however, and particularly since the work of Marcé[17], efforts were made to identify a separate brain pathology for senile dementia, in subjects who had not previously suffered from mental illness. Research in this group became important because it avoided the problem of having to decide whether or not the brain lesions were related to primary states of mania or melancholia. By the early 1900s, attempts had also been made to measure the symptoms and severity of dementia[11,14,18], to ascertain the differential importance of its senile and vascular aetiologies[19,20], and to study the frequency of senile dementia in relation to other psychiatric disorders affecting the elderly[21-23]. These enquiries were influenced by current theories on the ageing of brain tissue, such as that by Marinesco[24], who proposed that it started in the neurons.

Up to half a century earlier, brain changes believed to be associated with psychiatric disease were described in the language of gross anatomy[25,26]; they involved alterations in colour, consistency, weight, volume, and the relative proportion of solids to fluids. These observations, though, like all early microscopic work, were hampered by inadequate preserving, fixing, and staining techniques—staining artifacts in particular. Yet at the end of the century, the Cambridge anatomist Hardy considered it 'one of the most remarkable facts in the history of biological science that the urgency and priority of this question should have appealed to so few minds'[27].

But what was 'seen' also depended upon what theory the observer was using[28]. Agreement was needed not only on shapes and colours, but also on what they meant, what structures these features represented, and on what 'code of the body' was assumed[29]. After the 1890s, though, staining techniques improved in quality, and such animal studies as those by Ramón y Cajal[30] allowed a better understanding of the relationship between the resolution power of microscopes and putative lesions[31]. Alzheimer himself contributed to the development of staining methods, but his descriptions of pathological changes, like everyone else's in his time, were hampered by the fact that there was no general agreement on what the 'units of change', such as neurons or glia, really looked like. Nicolás Achúcarro, the talented Spanish pathologist who died very young, showed in Alzheimer's own laboratory that glial cells could give rise to formations which mimicked neurofibrillary tangles[32]. When Spielmeyer published his classic work on staining techniques[33], more than 100 had become available, of which about 15 were dedicated to making neurofibrils visible.

So far as the concept of the neuron was concerned, two views vied for supremacy between 1880 and the First World War. According to the neuronal theory, which had Ramón y Cajal as its champion, neurons were to be considered as independent units, never touching each other or doing so only sporadically. Reticularism, on the other hand, held that brain cells formed a 'syncitium'—a network of cells—and its leading figure was Golgi[34,35]. Waldeyer is recognized as having coined the term 'neurone' in 1891, although it may already have been used by Wilder[27]. The first round of the debate was won by the neuronists, but early in the twentieth century, Held, Bethe, and Apáthy revived a version of the reticularist view, the latter two also playing an important role in the discovery of neurofibrils[36]. These structures, significant in the later definition of some forms of senile dementia, were central to the reticularism debate.

Alzheimer's position on neuronal theory is unclear, although Nissl, his life-long friend, was in fact a reticularist[36,37].

Yet enquiries into the pathological changes which might accompany dementia had started early in the previous century, with descriptions of the appearance of the brain in subjects who had died in that state[26]. Both the variety of the changes and their non-specificity, though, made it difficult to reach any meaningful conclusion about them. In 1822, Bayle had described more or less recognizable abnormalities affecting the arachnoid in subjects showing both motor and psychological symptoms (including dementia). This encouraged the view that all manner of psychiatric disorders might also be related to brain pathology[25].

After the 1850s, efforts were made to separate out a sub-category of 'vesanic dementias', which included terminal states of the functional psychoses. For Marcé, cortical atrophy, enlarged ventricles, and tissue 'softening' became the macroscopic hallmark of 'senile dementia'[17]. The view that brain 'softening' was caused by changes in blood vessels was soon corroborated[38], but recognition of the distinction between vascular and parenchymal factors had to wait until the early twentieth century. From the 1880s, microscopic descriptions of such brains started to appear, and three changes were singled out as important: cellular death and disintegration, plaques, and neurofibrils; Beljahow reported in 1887 that the cells 'seemed to be broken down into formless clumps' (p262)[39]. Plaques were described in 1882 by Blocq and Marinesco (a great Rumanian histologist) in the brain of an epileptic patient, while Redlich re-described them in two elderly epileptics, and called them 'miliar sclerosis'[40,41].

However, the events that led to and immediately followed the first description of Alzheimer's disease, like the boundaries of the original description, are not easy to identify. The writings of Alzheimer, Fischer, Fuller, Lafora, Bonfiglio, Perusini, Ziveri, Kraepelin, and other major figures of the time are so deceptively fresh that reading them without taking today's view is difficult. And yet the psychiatry of the late nineteenth century is a remote country: as described above, even crucial concepts such as neuron, neurofibril, or plaque had not yet been fully crystallised, meaning different things then to different people. In fact, the mirage caused by a backward view from today can only be dispelled by exploring fully the history of the terms and issues that played the 'supporting cast' to the concept of Alzheimer's disease. These also include dementia, ageing, senile psychosis, and cerebral arteriosclerosis as well as methods of visualising brain tissue, the state of academic psychiatry, and university rivalries. Through such a process, it may be possible to reconstruct the perception that alienists of Alzheimer's time had of the disease.

One also has to ask what clinical problem was the 'creator' of a new entity trying to solve. In this case, Alzheimer seems to have been mainly interested in the early onset of the condition, its uncommon severity, its focal symptoms, and the simultaneous presence of plaques and tangles. But, if that is so, why was it *these* features, and not the simultaneous presence of arteriosclerotic changes, or of hallucinations and delusions that concerned him? One answer is that the major scientific debates of the time in this field were not about creating homogeneous diagnoses. They were rather about the foundations of neurobiology: whether neurons were independent units, whether they were capable of amoeboid movements[42,43], whether staining techniques were reliable, etc.

By Alzheimer's period, the organic dementias of the elderly had undergone classification into simple, complicated, and arteriosclerotic forms. Psychotic and other non-cognitive symptoms were a defining feature of the 'complicated dementias', and were the main reason for classifying dementia as an 'exogenous psychosis'[44-46]. What is more, the meaning of the various psychotic symptoms also changed over time. Originally, they were classified as objective (action disorders) or subjective (experiential), and both were believed to carry equal diagnostic weight: among the former, disorders of movement such as catalepsy, catatonia, and mannerisms sometimes took diagnostic precedence. This was due to the fact that movement disorders were believed to reflect specific organic impairments, and is well illustrated by the work of Kahlbaum and of Wernicke, as well as in Kraepelinian and Bleulerian psychopathology.

After the First World War, however, a shift in the emphasis of diagnosis took place, starting with the work of Mayer Gross and culminating in that of Schneider. For both theoretical reasons (as with Freud) and 'empirical reasons' (as with Schneider), subjective or 'experiential' symptoms became central to the diagnosis of schizophrenia: auditory hallucinations, passivity feelings, and delusions were then more important than the motor disorders. This change worked well in the case of schizophrenia, since it increased the reliability of diagnosis; generally, schizophrenics have no cognitive impairment and can describe their experience. But it is otherwise in the case of dementia, where experiential symptoms are particularly difficult to verify, and this may be an important reason for the neglect of psychotic symptoms in this disorder.

In the 1990s, Alzheimer and his disease have become the flavour of the decade: books, a dedicated Journal, and a large number of research papers attest to this fact. Clinicians increasingly face demands from basic scientists to provide subjects for research studies who meet 'strict DSM III-R diagnostic criteria' of the disorder. The race between pharmaceutical companies to find the 'cure' for Alzheimer's disease is fierce, and established scientists have been recruited to the task. Yet all this activity surrounds a disease which until the Second World War was considered infrequent, judging by the epidemiological estimates of the period and the few publications devoted to it. So has there been a sudden increase in the incidence and prevalence of Alzheimer's disease which is not simply a consequence of ageing populations? Is the prediction of a 'silent epidemic'[47] becoming a reality? Historians of science tell us that shifts in scientific fashion are never simple affairs, and that social and ideological reasons must be sought for them[2,48-50]. How is it that from being one amongst many degenerative diseases affecting the elderly, this condition has become so 'common'?

'Primary degenerative dementia of the Alzheimer type' is defined in DSM III-R as a dementia of insidious onset with a 'generally progressive, deteriorating course for which all other specific causes have been excluded by the history, physical examination, and laboratory tests. The dementia involves a multifaceted loss of intellectual abilities, such as memory, judgement, abstract thought, and other higher cortical functions, and changes in personality and behaviour' (pp119-120)[48]. Like all definitions by exclusion, the sensitivity of this one is a function of the sharpness of instruments and tests, and of clinical knowledge on all the other types of dementia. It is not surprising, therefore, that in this case the diagnostic sensitivity and specificity, particularly in cross-sectional studies, are not satisfactory[49,50]. This definition seems also to assume that Alzheimer's disease is a unitary condition, separable from 'senile dementia'. Studies, however, suggest that there are subgroupings such as an autosomal dominant, familial, and sporadic types[51], or AD1 and AD2 groups, the latter occurring early, and having a rampant course and more impairment of parietal lobe and locus coeruleus[52]—this classification has been adopted by ICD-10[53]. There may even be four groups: benign, myoclonic, extrapyramidal and typical[54], or the assumption of discontinuity from senile dementia may be unwarranted[55]. Although differentiable on a statistical basis, the subgroups described show much overlap and cannot be reliably used for diagnostic purposes[56].

The fundamental problem is that in spite of the large amount of completed research[57], not enough is known on any one specific feature of the disease to develop a valid marker. The cholinergic hypothesis has not lived up to its early promise[58] and genetic studies have been equally disappointing, in spite of the exciting discovery that the proximal segment of the long arm of chromosome 21[59] may include loci for Alzheimer's disease, Down's syndrome, and the A4 amyloid gene. Static neuroimaging has probably reached the limits of its usefulness, although atrophy of the hyppocampi may be an early marker[60]. Functional techniques, such as PET, SPECT, and EEG brain mapping have shown some striking changes (e.g. those incriminating parieto-temporal areas)[61], but the usefulness of these findings in clinical practice remains undetermined. Neuropsychological efforts to identify a 'typical' profile of cognitive deficit have not yet come to fruition, and no agreed battery of tests has emerged[62], though this should not be surprising in view of the fact that we still lack a unified model of memory.

So paradoxically, the more that scientific detail has accumulated on Alzheimer's disease, the more elusive the 'illness' has become. In an effort to make it a separate entity, the creators of the disease may have narrowed its clinical boundaries unduly, so that current research workers are trapped in the vicious circle of only finding what they have themselves put there in the first place. It is perhaps time, therefore, to take a longer look at the historical evolution of these concepts, and we hope that this book will contribute to this endeavour. The history of Alzheimer's disease, like that of the other dementias, has been neglected until recently[63-66]. One reason for this has been the fact that crucial material was untranslated or difficult to obtain, but Bick et al have now helped English-speaking scholars who are without knowledge of the German and Italian languages by offering renditions of six crucial papers[67,68], and Förstl and Levy have done likewise with Alzheimer's all-important 1911 paper[69]. Yet more needs to be done in other areas, for example, on the social history and dynamics of Alzheimer's own department, on the contribution of visiting scientists such as Perusini, Lafora, Achúcarro, and Fuller, and on the views and contributions of Oskar Fischer and the Prague school.

Likewise, not much has until recently been known about Alois Alzheimer himself. There is even disagreement as to the extent of his clinical interests. Hippius has suggested that they were very strong, and that all he really wanted to do was to look after patients[70]. On the other hand, visitors to his department described him as a shy person, who was at his happiest when looking down a microscope. As shown by the list appended to Hoff's chapter, it would seem that he was interested in various diseases, and even in the theoretical aspects of psychiatry. For example, he had a debate with Alfred Hoche on the question of how best to conceptualise mental illness, and criticised Wernicke (who at the time was already dead) in respect of his overstated localisationism. It would be an exaggeration, however, to say, that Alzheimer was an original thinker in this field for, as Hippius has shown, he faithfully followed the views of Kraepelin, and it is likely that he was less aware than Kraepelin was of the importance of social and political variables on scientific thinking. This might explain why he felt reluctant to accept his chief's view that the syndrome he had described constituted, in fact, a new disease.

It is hoped that the succeeding chapters on Alzheimer himself, on the dementias, and on the clinical, social, and cultural issues surrounding them, will throw useful light on the various issues mentioned above, and will help to increase understanding of this major scourge of mankind.

Chapter 2

Dementia Before the Twentieth Century

G. E. Berrios and H. L. Freeman

Attempts at elucidating the history of dementia before the nine-teenth century have not been very successful so far, since the history of the word itself has not been separated from those of the concept and the behavioural phenomena to which it should relate. One problem is that this term was often used to refer to states quite different from what is currently called dementia. 'Dementia' can be found as early as the Latin works of Lucretius, where its central sense was simply that of 'being out of one's mind'[1], but at various times, words such as amentia, imbecility, morosis, fatuitas, foolish-ness, stupidity, anoea, simplicity, carus, idiocy, dotage, and seni-lity were also used to describe conditions of intellectual and behavioural deterioration.

Thomas Willis (1684) included states of dementia under the category 'Stupidity, or Foolishness', which 'athough it mostly chiefly belongs to the rational soul, and signifies a defect of the intellect and judgement, yet it is not improperly reckoned among the diseases of the head or brain; for as much as this eclipse of the superior soul proceeds from the imagination and the memory being hurt, and the failing of these depends upon the faults of the animal spirits, and the brain itself' (p209)[2]. Willis suggested that stupidity could be either 'original' (as when 'fools beget fools') or acquired by ageing ('Some at first crafty and ingenious, become by degrees dull, and at length foolish, by the mere declining of age, without any great errors in living') (p211), or by 'strokes or bruising upon the head', 'drunkenness and surfeiting', 'violent and sudden passions' and 'cruel diseases of the head' such as epilepsy.

THE EIGHTEENTH CENTURY

The earliest usage in English of 'demented' is dated by the Oxford English Dictionary (OED) to 1644, while 'dementia' appears in the vernacular in Blancard's popular *Physical Dictionary* (1726)[3], where it was considered as equivalent to 'anoea' or 'extinction of the imagination and judgment' (p21). It has not yet been found in earlier dictionaries[4-6], though the Latin stem 'demens' (without mind) seems to have been incorporated into the vernaculars of Western Europe sometime during the seventeenth century. Evidence of definitive use can be found in the *Encyclopédie ou Dictionnaire Raisonné de Sciences, des Arts et des Métières* (French Encyclopaedia) (1765)[7]. The OED refers the earliest usage in English of 'dementia' to Davis's translation of Pinel's *Treatise of Insanity*: where it was said to be 'first used to render the term *démence de Pinel*'[8], though the term was not actually coined by Pinel, who first used it to translate Cullen's work in his *Institutiones de Médicine-Pratique*[9]. Sobrino's classical Spanish-French dictionary gave a clear definition in 1791: 'demencia: démence, folie, extravagance, egarement, alienation d'sprit' (p300)[10]. During that century, the term acquired a medical connotation, and began to mean any states of impaired psychosocial competence, whether congenital or acquired, temporary or permanent, and affecting the young or the old.

In the **French Encyclopaedia**, the long entry on *démence* may have been written by Arnulfe d'Aumont[11], Professor of Medicine at Valence. It has two parts (medical and legal); the medical section (in our translation) states that:

'Dementia is a disease consisting in a paralysis of the spirit characterised by an abolition of the reasoning faculty. It differs from fatuitas, morosis, stultitia and stoliditas in that in the latter there is a diminution or weakening of understanding and memory; and from delirium in that in the latter there is only an impairment in ... the said functions. Those affected by dementia exhibit foolish behaviour and cannot understand what they are told, cannot remember anything, have no judgment, are sluggish, and retarded.

Abolition [of subjective experiences] may result from: 1. damage to the brain caused by excessive usage, congenital causes or old age, 2. failure of the spirit, 3. small volume of the brain, 4. violent blows to the head causing brain damage, 5. incurable diseases such as epilepsy, or exposure to venoms ...

Dementia is difficult to cure as it is probably related to damage of brain fibres or of nervous fluids. Dementia is incurable if it is associated with a congenital defect or with old age ... this disease is therefore always chronic, continuous ... if it follows sadness or tiredness of the mind it can be made better by rest and entertainment ... shepherds and butchers, have observed that sheep can develop a form of dementia during which they refuse to eat or drink ... their brains being often reduced to almost nothing or to a serosity' [this seems to be an early reference to scrapie].

The legal section reads:

> 'Those who are in a state of dementia are incapable of informed
> consent, cannot enter into contracts, sign wills, or be members
> of a jury . . . they are declared as incapable of managing their
> own affairs. Actions carried out before the declaration of incapa-
> city, however, are valid unless it can be demonstrated that
> the dementia had anteceded these actions. Evidence for a state
> of dementia must be based on a close examination of the writings
> of these individuals, answers during interview by magistrates and
> doctors, and the testimony of others.[1]

These entries, written by a physician without any special interest
in 'psychiatry', reflect middle-of-the-road views of the late eighteenth
century. For the educated man, then, dementia was both a medical
and a legal state, the medical definition being based on psychosocial
competence, with little mention of accompanying symptoms such
as behavioural disorder. Dementia was clearly distinguished from
'mania' (a term which at the time described states of excitement,
whether schizophrenic, hypomanic, or organic) and from 'delirium'
(which referred more or less to the present 'acute confusional state').
It affected individuals of any age, including the elderly, and tended
to be chronic and irreversible (mainly in the elderly), although
irreversibility was not an essential feature. The reference to
congenital or acquired brain lesions, drug-induced states, sadness
(depression), and epilepsy as causes is important, suggesting that
the syndromal view of dementia had already developed during this
period and not during the early nineteenth century.

The legal meaning was to become central to Article 10 of the
Napoleonic Code (1810)[12]: 'There is no crime if the accused was in
a state of dementia at the time of the alleged act', though this usage
was not specific to French law. Hale in England had already
distinguished (in the middle of the seventeenth century) between
dementia naturalis, *accidentalis*, and *affectata*, according to whether
the intellectual incompetence was congenital, or due to mental illness
or 'toxic disorders'[13]. However, the defining features of dementia
that were to develop fully during the nineteenth century can already
be found here: a disorder of the intellectual functions that led to
behavioural incapacity, its duration depending on the cause, which
could be either an organic or a 'functional' disorder, and this either
congenital or acquired.

Cullen and the states of 'Amentia'
Description of the behavioural syndrome currently called 'dementia'
during the eighteenth century as 'amentia' culminated in the work
of Cullen (1712-1790), the great Edinburgh physician who first
coined the term 'neuroses'. He had based his disease classification

on clinical observation, but was using the principles of 'neuralpathology'—the view that all diseases were, in the last instance, diseases of the nervous system[14]. Nonetheless, Cullen simplified the over-inflated classifications of his predecessors, defining the 'neuroses' as diseases without fever whose central feature was a putative non-localised disturbance of 'sense and motion' in the nervous system. These wide, theoretical criteria allowed him to bring together a large number of syndromes within the class 'neuroses' (of which the 'vesanias', i.e. the insanities, were one order); they were further defined as resulting from pathological changes in the status of an invisible (Newtonian) fluid. He defined 'amentia' as a loss of intellectual functions and memory, and divided it into congenital, senile, and acquired forms; the causes for the latter included infections, vascular disorders, sexual excesses, poisons, and trauma. In this way, Cullen distinguished states of mental retardation from those of senile dementia and from those related to brain damage of various causes[15]. When Pinel translated Cullen's nosology into French, he used the term 'dementia' throughout.

Pinel

The old view that Pinel was the first alienist of the nineteenth century can no longer be sustained; by ideology and temperament, he was, in fact, the last great nosologist of the eighteenth. Descriptions of states of dementia appear often in his writings, but under other terms. In the *Nosographie*, for example, he included them under the categories of 'amentia' and 'morosis', and described them in behavioural terms: failure in the association of ideas, disordered activity, extravagant behaviour, superficial emotions, memory loss, difficulty in the perception of objects, obliteration of judgment, aimless activity, automatic existence, and forgetting words or signs[16]. He also referred to *démence senile* (para 116), thus disproving Cohen's point (1983) that 'the term senile dementia was first used by Esquirol' (p30)[17], and included sections on the differential diagnosis (118), aetiology (119) and treatment (121) of dementia.

Following Willis and Cullen, Pinel did not feel the need to consider states of congenital and acquired dementia as different diseases. Esquirol's poetic suggestion (*vide infra*) as to how idiocy and dementia were to be distinguished was only possible after the relevance of congenital states to idiocy had been discussed in French psychiatry, in the wake of Itard's account of the Wild Boy of Aveyron. There is little evidence, however, for Mahendra's suggestion (p9)[18] that general socioeconomic factors may also have favoured the distinction between idiocy and dementia.

Pinel acted as the link between eighteenth- and nineteenth-century views on dementia; through him, the term and concept became well established to include all states of psychosocial incompetence due to impairment of intellectual function. These could be reversible or irreversible, congenital or acquired, and caused by brain disorder or by insanity. Towards 1900, however, 'dementia' was being used to refer to specific states of cognitive impairment, mostly irreversible and mainly affecting the elderly. Meanwhile, after a period of disuse, 'amentia' had re-appeared as the term for a 'psychosis, with sudden onset following severe, often acute physical illness or trauma'[19]. Many great writers, influenced by changing views on psychological theory and neuropathology, made the process whereby the concept of dementia was narrowed down, eventually leading to a view compatible with what Kraepelin was to call Alzheimer's disease. Their views will be surveyed briefly as the background to the main theme of this book.

DEMENTIA DURING THE NINETEENTH CENTURY

FRENCH VIEWS

Esquirol
Though there have been claims that Esquirol's views on dementia were more advanced than those of Pinel[20], his usage, in fact, varied a great deal: in *Des passions* (1805)[21], he repeatedly used the word in a general way (*démence accidental*, *démence mélancolique*, etc.) to refer to temporary changes in cognitive function or to loss of reason. In 1814, for the 'Panckouke' dictionary, he distinguished between acute, chronic, and senile dementia, as well as suggesting a 'composite' type which included the dementia associated with melancholia, mania, epilepsy, convulsions, scurvy, and paralysis. Acute dementia was a short-lived state, was reversible, and followed fevers, haemorrhages, metastasis, and the mental weakness caused by mania. Chronic dementia tended to be irreversible and might be caused by masturbation, melancholia, mania, hypochondria, epilepsy, paralysis, and apoplexy, while senile dementia resulted from ageing, and consisted in a loss of the faculties of understanding[22].

Meanwhile, in 1826, Bayle published his work on diseases of the brain, embodying a more anatomical or organic view of the insanities. For instance, in general paralysis of the insane, whilst Bayle suggested that the brain changes caused both the mental and motor symptoms, Esquirol and his group claimed that it was the insanity itself which led to the paralysis. What was at stake was whether dementia was a primary or a secondary state[23].

In 1838, Esquirol reported 15 cases of dementia with a mean age of 34 years (sd=10.9)! There were seven males and eight females, and the diagnoses included seven cases of general paralysis of the insane—showing a combination of grandiosity, disinhibition, motor symptoms, dysarthria, and terminal cognitive failure; on post-mortem, five had arachnoiditis. There was also a 20 year-old girl with a catatonic syndrome (in our present diagnosis), showing alternating stupor and excitement and eventual recovery, who was diagnosed as 'acute dementia', as well as a 40 year-old woman with pica and cognitive impairment who was found to have two space-occupying lesions[24]. The choice of these patients by Esquirol as illustrations is interesting, particularly in the absence of any with senile dementia, which often appears in early nineteenth-century classifications as an afterthought. The same was true of irreversibility; this only became a criterion when the vesanic dementias (i.e. states of defect caused by chronic psychoses) were eliminated from the classification. Esquirol's contribution consisted mainly in the reorganisation of the syndrome in terminological, classificatory, and anatomo-pathological terms, in response to changes in the philosophy of medicine.

Georget

During his short life (1795-1828), Georget wrote two important books including *De la Folie*, published when he was only 25, which offered a more dynamic approach to the description and classification of mental disorders[25]. He contributed to the consolidation of the concept of stupidity or stupor[26], which Esquirol still called 'acute dementia'. Generalising from his neuropathological work, Georget suggested that all mental disorders depended on diseases of the brain. He disagreed with Esquirol's claim that the cognitive impairment found in subjects with dementia was due to a primary deficit of attention, suggesting that it was a reversible state. He recognised two irreversible states, idiocy and dementia, claiming that in both there was an abolition of thought; the first originated from a 'vice' in the organisation of the brain, and the second from weakening, old age, or intercurrent diseases (p37).

Georget's views on dementia are a reflection of his general conception of mental illness. He criticised 'great men' such as Pinel, Esquirol, Crichton, Perfect, Haslam, Chiaruggi, and Rush for being too fearful of contradicting philosophical or religious beliefs, and describing mental illness: 'without touching upon causes, and considering the disorders of function without referring to the organs that supported them . . . giving the impression that it was the symptoms that constituted the illness and not the corresponding organic lesion' (ppvii-viii). This organicism led him to postulate a narrow and modern-sounding concept of dementia, as well as raising the issue of irreversibility.

Calmeil

Far more aware than Esquirol or Georget of the problems involved in the clinical description of mental disorder, Calmeil wrote in

1835 that 'it is not easy to describe dementia, its varieties, and nuances . . . nor its distinctive symptoms' (p71)[27]. Dementia might follow chronic insanity or brain disease, and could be partial and general; he was less convinced that all cases were associated with gross brain change. So far as the pathological substratum was concerned, he believed there was not sufficient information on the nature and range of anomalies found in the skull or brain to decide which were causes of and which were caused by dementia (pp82-83).

Guislain

Guislain's two main works were *Traité sur la Alienation Mental* (1826)[28] and his *Lectures*, published in 1852. Dementia appears as the third class of his classification (p10)[29], defined in opposition to mania:

> 'all intellectual functions show a marked reduction in their energy, external stimuli cause only minor impression in the intellect, imagination is not only weak but uncreative, memory is almost totally absent, and reasoning is pathological . . . There are two varieties . . . . one affecting the elderly (senile dementia of Cullen) and another acquired earlier in life . . . idiocy must be considered as a separate group'.

Guislain offered what may well be the earliest version of an operational definition of 'cognitive failure', when describing a clear case of dementia:

> 'The patient has no memory, or at least is unable to retain anything that was told him, all impressions evaporate from his mind. He may occasionally remember the names of people but not if he has met or seen them before. He . . . has lost the instinct of preservation, and thus cannot avoid fire or water and is unable to recognize dangers; has lost all spontaneity, is incontinent of urine and faeces, he does not ask for anything, he is impassive and cannot recognize his wife or children' (p311).

Guislain's main contribution was to identify diagnostic criteria, which included orientation tests, as well as behavioural elements that served to stage the progress of the state of dementia.

Marc

In 1840, CCH Marc published *On insanity and its Relationship to Medico-legal Issues*, a classical forensic psychiatry treatise which was to remain influential for many years. 'In legal language', he wrote 'the word dementia is considered as tantamount to insanity; in medical language, however, it names only one of the forms of insanity' (p261)[30]. The main legal 'criteria' included weakness of the understanding and of the will, as well as loss of memory and of judgment. Marc believed that doctors found great difficulty in making a diagnosis in five clinical situations: early dementia, i.e. when some mental faculties are well preserved; sudden onset, when no prodromal features can be found; when 'lucid intervals' are present; when the state of dementia is accompanied by hallucinations and delusions; and in malingering. He was very aware of the need to integrate the medical and legal meanings, and clearly identified some of the difficulties that expert witnesses had to face in Court. Similar moves were occurring in Germany, as attested by the work of Hoffbauer (*vide infra*, section on Germany).

Morel
Morel, better known for his views on 'degeneration theory', was in fact a great clinician and classificator, and his views on dementia constitute a landmark in the French psychiatric scene. His role in European psychiatry was crucial to the development of the modern nosology of mental illness. Morel's classification of mental disorders respected the 'close and necessary relationship existing between their form [i.e. the symptoms] and their cause'. Thus, six groups were identified: hereditary, toxic, resulting from the transformation of neuroses, idiopathic, sympathetic, and the dementias. Suggesting that the dementias are mostly 'terminal states', Morel wrote that while there are: 'Exceptional individuals who until the end will preserve plenitude of their intellectual faculties . . . the majority are subject to the law of decline of faculties. This law follows the loss of vitality in the brain; chronic cases [of insanity] tend to show general impairment of intelligence (dementia). This weight decrement, a constant feature of dementia, is also the natural result of ageing, and of the decadence that characterized the human species'[31].

He distinguished two types: 'natural dementia and that resulting from a pathological state of the brain . . . some forms of insanity are proner to end up in dementia (idiopathic)' (pp837-838). Morel's views were novel in that he applied his own evolutionary and degenerationist concepts, which made the dementias just terminal stages for most, if not all mental illness. But this necessitated the assumption that to develop dementia, all subjects had to go through some form of insanity. To explain the many cases in which no history of mental illness was found, he resorted to two explanatory notions— ageing and degeneration. This view of dementia as a terminal state also dissuaded Morel from seeking a specific form of brain pathology for senile dementia.

GERMAN VIEWS
At the beginning of the nineteenth century, German writings on alienism were, with few exceptions, little known and hence

uninfluential in both France and England. Alexander Crichton included in his *Inquiry* (1798)[32] some case vignettes and ideas he had taken from the journal edited by Charles Philip Moritz and Salomon Maimon—the first psychiatric periodical in the world. However, the Kantian ideas on which this publication was based remained unknown further afield until in 1811, on his return from Germany, Coleridge lectured about them in England.[33] In general, though, no influence of German psychiatric ideas on other European countries can be detected up to the 1840s.

Heinroth

Heinroth published more than 35 books, but his contribution has not yet been fully elucidated; the conventional view sees him as a spiritualist physician who believed that 'mental illness was a sin', but this view is almost certainly mistaken[34]. In his *Textbook*, clinical states suggesting dementia were described as complications of mental disorders resulting from functional exaltations or depressions of the mind. The former gave rise to 'mania' (a condition still described in the old sense of acute, raging insanity) and to dementia if the disorder continued for a long time: 'the intellect will be thrown overboard, and the morbid state becomes habitual' (p163). The 'patient appears to be sane, except for his understanding and judgement' (p169)[35]. 'Melancholia' (also defined in its old sense of retarded insanity—and not of mental depression) was itself caused by a decline in mental functioning, and if prolonged might lead to idiocy and apathy. Both could also give rise to states of reversible stupor, and less commonly to longer lasting states of cognitive impairment; when they were combined, subjects often developed chronic confusion.

Hoffbauer

Early in the nineteenth century, *Blödsinn* and *Dummheit* were more or less the equivalent German terms to the French *démence*, and the English 'dementia'; *Blödsinn* referred to chronic and mostly irreversible states, and *Dummheit* to acute, reversible forms of dementia[36]. The chronic group, in turn, was divided by Hoffbauer into senile dementia (always incurable) and the secondary dementias, which were the final or defect state of various forms of mental illness and only rarely curable. This latter group was equivalent to the French 'vesanic dementias'.

Translated by the French alienist AM Chambeyron, Hoffbauer's text also carried clarificatory but often critical footnotes by Esquirol and Itard. Regarding Hoffbauer's suggestion that there were many varieties of mental weakness, a footnote reads: 'all the distinctions established by the author between stupidity and imbecility are unintelligible to French readers. In fact, the differences expressed are just degrees of dementia' (p60).

Feuchtersleben

Hoffbauer's broad definition of dementia remained alive in German-speaking psychiatry until the 1840s, but in his *Textbook of Medical Psychology*[37], Feuchtersleben considered this category tantamount to 'insanity'. Indeed, the English translator of the book used the term 'folly' to render Feuchtersleben's *Blödsinn*[38]. This Austrian physician also provides a glimpse of what a technical description of senile dementia might have been like before the development of the cognitive paradigm—the idea that memory decline was the central symptom of dementia[39]. He made senile dementia equivalent to a state of idiocy occurring in the elderly, and defined it as an 'incapacity of judging, or even, in its higher degree, of contemplating. The alteration is more prominent in the direction of thought than in that of feeling and will, though in the higher degrees, both feelings and will are also wanting' (p301). Consistent with his view, Feuchtersleben did not even mention senile dementia in the section of the book on the memory disorders, where all other mnesic deficits were treated in detail (pp237-240).

Griesinger

Griesinger broke away from the classical views of Hoffbauer, and put forward a new notion of dementia; he had a rather irreverent attitude to the old classifications. Surprisingly in a man who did not have much clinical experience, he tried to reject clinical definitions which included much theory. However, his model of mental illness was still based on the view that each psychological function might be exalted, depressed, or weakened, and that each functional state gave rise to a different type of mental illness. He believed that although brain disease was at the basis of all mental disorders, their full understanding required social and psychological factors to be also taken into consideration.

This led Griesinger to sponsor, in his book of 1861, a modified form of 'unitary' psychosis according to which mania, melancholia, and dementia were three successive stages of the same basic insanity. This model allowed him to define dementia in a new fashion, and to identify at least five varieties of mental disorder in which there was a weakening of mental faculties: chronic mania, dementia, apathetic dementia, idiocy, and cretinism. Dementia was included in the states of mental weakness not showing delusions, but distinguished from apathetic dementia:

'the fundamental disorder consists in a general weakness of the mental faculties. Increasing incapacity for any profound emotion, loss of memory, and (reduced) power of reproduction of ideas . . . more recent events . . . are almost immediately forgotten, while not infrequently former ideas connected with events which happened long ago are more easily reproduced . . . complete remissions never occur' (pp340-343)[40].

However this recalls current descriptions of senile dementia, Griesinger was talking about a terminal mental state which constituted the third stage of insanity, occurring at any age of life and after an illness that currently might be called mania, schizophrenia, or organic disorder. His notion of 'apathetic dementia' is less well defined, although 'senile dementia' was included as one of its subtypes. Like other writers of this period, he did not distinguish primary degeneration of the brain from vascular damage as causes of senility.

Krafft-Ebing
In 1876, Krafft-Ebing[41] suggested that it was important to separate states of insanity affecting the elderly, which behaved as in earlier life and hence were reversible, from senile dementia, which was a disease that specifically affected old age, though it was not easy to decide what age ought to be the cut-off point. When there were intercurrent diseases, 50 might be a reasonable limit, but senile dementia rarely occurred spontaneously before 65. He believed that heredity and other external causes were far less important to the development of senile dementia than the natural changes accompanying ageing, including poor cerebral nutrition, anaemia, atheroma, and degeneration of the cortical cells. Clinically, demented patients were distractable, vacant, repetitious, disorientated, showed loss of memory, and could no longer recognise family members or places that were once familiar to them. As the dementia progressed, patients might show states of mania or melancholia, punctuated by hallucinations, paranoid delusions, fear of being robbed, etc. In 1888, in the third edition of his *Textbook*[42], Krafft-Ebing dedicated a full section to senile dementia (pp689-695).

Kraepelin
Kraepelin changed his mind about senile dementia a number of times. In the first edition of his *Lectures* (1904)[43], he dealt with 'senile imbecility' as one of the disorders of old age. After discussing melancholia and persecutory states, he reported the case of a shoemaker who had had his neck broken and afterwards developed an agitated depression, severe hypochondriacal delusions, and, in addition, 'a pronounced inability to retain new mental impressions' (p223) associated with 'a good memory concerning ideas formed long ago'. Recognition of these cases was important, as 'senile imbecility is of its very nature incurable, since it depends on the destruction of several constituents of the cortex'. Though depression or excitement might occur at first, 'the end will always be a high degree of mental and emotional feebleness' (pp223-224). In the second

edition, the corresponding chapter was entitled 'Senile Dementia', and three clinical illustrations were given, though one of them was, in fact, a case of depressive stupor[44].

Finally, in the 1909 edition of his *Textbook*[45], Kraepelin dealt separately with pre-senile and senile dementia. In the section on senile dementia, Kraepelin discussed the psychological changes of old age and concluded that 'in the most serious cases', these alterations themselves led to 'the disease pattern of dementia' (p593). He described the typical cognitive and memory impairment, changes in personality and emotions, and the brain abnormalities associated with senile dementia. He also mentioned the description by Alzheimer of a 'particular group of cases with extremely serious cell alterations', and the naming of the disease. 'The clinical interpretation of this *Alzheimer's disease* is still confused. While the anatomical findings suggest that one is dealing with a particular serious form of senile dementia, the fact that this disease sometimes starts already around the age of 40 does not allow this supposition. In such cases we should at least assume a 'senium praecox', *if not perhaps a more or less age-independent unique disease process*' (pp627-628).

Ziehen

Parallel to the synthetic work of Kraepelin on dementia was the classification of Theodor Ziehen, one of the most original German alienists of the period. He was well aware of the difficulties involved in the notion of vesanic dementia and of the research findings showing characteristic structural changes only in some groups of 'dementia', particularly in old age. With minor changes, his classification was to last up to the Second World War; it contained nine groups of dementia, in the following order of importance: senile, arteriosclerotic, apoplectic (focal), post-meningitic, toxic (post-alcoholic, lead intoxication, etc.), traumatic, secondary to functional psychoses (vesanic), epileptic, and hebephrenic or praecox. He defined senile dementia as 'mental disease affecting old age characterised by a progressive weakening of intellectual faculties and caused by cortical involution (without the intervention of causes such as alcohol or syphilis)' (p282)[46]. The involution of the grey matter was said to affect neurons and fibres directly, but blood vessels only occasionally. He believed that dementias starting before 60 reflected states of 'praecox senility', and that these were hereditary in origin. Generalised arteriosclerosis, often affecting the heart, could also accompany some dementias, as could a history of head trauma, but overwork was dismissed as an irrelevant factor.

Memory failure, particularly affecting recent events, was for Ziehen the hallmark of senile dementia, interpreted as a defect in the formation of associations; general intellectual and affective deterioration and the presence of hallucinations and delusions were also important symptoms. This led him to describe both a 'simple' form of senile dementia (characterised only by cognitive impairment) and a complex one (accompanied by psychotic and affective symptoms), which might be confused with the stuporous forms of melancholia (p299). From the pathological point of view, Ziehen limited himself to enumerating 13 putative brain changes, but only Alzheimer's earlier reports were cited. He did not have anything to say on what Kraepelin had two years earlier called 'Alzheimer's disease'.

Jaspers
Jaspers first wrote on dementia in a paper dealing with both the concept and the psychometric techniques available at the time to measure 'intelligence'[47]. The crucial feature of dementia was that it was 'permanent'; he suggested that the methods developed to measure intelligence in the normal person should be used to assess cognitive decline. Jaspers quoted Kraepelin's definition of dementia, but commented that 'It would seem that any failure in performance, whatever the way it is assessed, is called dementia. The concept, therefore, is so wide that, like other overencompassing notions, it is in danger of being almost empty of real content'. His own suggestion was that dementia should be diagnosed 'in any situation when there is an omission of any of the necessary constituents of cognition, and as a result a situation of false thinking can be identified'.

In the last edition of the *General Psychopathology* (1948)[48], Jaspers recommended the old psychometric tests of Ebbinghaus and Stern, as well as criteria to differentiate the various states in which intelligent behaviour may fail. One of these was the syndrome of 'organic dementia': 'the organic process usually destroys in a far-reaching manner the pre-conditions (*Vorbedingungen*) of intelligence, such as memory, powers of organisation, and sometimes the apparatus of speech, so that, for instance, in senile dementia . . . a person forgets his whole life, cannot speak properly any longer, and can make himself understood only with difficulty' (p184). Thus, Jaspers remained loyal to the idea that 'intelligent behaviour' constitutes a unitary form of activity whose failure will depend on how its various components are affected by disease. This association-istic approach, out of fashion for about 40 years, is now once again popular in the neuropsychiatry of dementia.

BRITISH VIEWS

Although 'dementia' can be found in English law since the seventeenth century, its medical usage only started early in the nineteenth; before this, clinical states of cognitive disorganisation, whether in the young or the old, were recognised but described differently. For example, Sir John Roberts of Bromley was described by William Salmon in 1694 as 'decayed in his intellectuals' (p778)[49], and D'Assingy (1706) noticed that in some 'cases it is impossible to remedy a decay'd memory' (p19)[50].

Prichard

With characteristic lucidity, the Bristol alienist Prichard wrote of dementia that: 'it may be thought scarcely correct to term this a form of insanity, as it has been generally considered as a result or sequel of the disease. In some instances, however, mental derangement has clearly this character from the commencement or at least assumes it at a very early period' (p6)[51]. Instead of 'a French term', he suggested 'incoherence', which he regarded as far more than mere breakdown in association of ideas—a popular theory then. Though referring to a gradual deterioration of the whole mental life, he treated senile dementia separately: 'it is entirely distinct from that species of moral insanity which appears occasionally . . . in aged persons. The former is merely a loss of energy in some of the intellectual functions . . . It is in senile decay that the phenomena of incoherence in the first degree (i.e. forgetfulness) are mostly strongly marked' (p93). In this, Prichard showed his common sense; he did not seem to have had a great deal of clinical experience and was relatively uninfluenced by theory.

Bucknill & Tuke

By the middle of the century, internal contradictions in the definition of the concept of dementia were more or less hidden by the deft use of classifications. In their *Manual* (1858), Bucknill & Tuke summarised the views of Pinel, Esquirol, Guislain, and Prichard: they described how patients with mania, melancholia, old age, etc. may develop dementia, and discussed the definitions and types. Memory loss must be a central symptom (p119), but dementia could be either: 'primary or consecutive . . . acute or chronic . . . simple or complicated . . . occasionally remittent but rarely intermittent' (p117)[52]. The acute form was rare, the chronic irreversible, and the senile 'another variety although when established it differs little in its symptoms from the chronic form' (p122).

Hughlings Jackson

Though a neurologist, Hughlings Jackson put forward some concepts and models which seem more relevant to mental than to neurological disorder. Yet he did not believe in 'mental' illness, and suggested that all the 'insanities', from the obsessional to the delusional states and the dementias, were simply the behavioural reflection of successive stages of the dismantling of cerebral structures—which Jackson called 'dissolution'. He believed these various layers of the brain had been deposited by evolution, and ranged from the most primitive, stable, and organised, to the more human, disorganised, and unstable. Since the top layers were assumed to inhibit the lower ones[53], diseases affected the top layers and in destroying them, obliterated their function (negative symptoms), while the lower structures tried to compensate, causing positive symptoms. On the effect of age, Jackson wrote: 'we rarely, if ever, meet with a dissolution from disease which is the exact reversal of evolution. Probably healthy senescence is the dissolution most nearly the exact reversal of evolution' (p413)[54]. The deepest form of dissolution, coma, he called 'acute temporary dementia: Let us say that the patient is, or is nearly, mentally dead' (p412). For Jackson, dementia was the only form of insanity without positive symptoms.

Jackson's treatment of dementia, like other mental disorders, was theoretical and related little to clinical practice. Though criticised by the alienists of his time, this model became influential later in French psychiatry. Julian de Ajurriaguerra[55] combined it with Piagetian ideas of development and suggested that in dementia, there is an ordered dismantling of layers which can explain the various serial syndromes observed in Alzheimer's disease, including the stage when the subject may exhibit hallucinations and delusions.

Maudsley

In *The Pathology of the Mind* (1879), Henry Maudsley included a chapter on 'Conditions of mental weakness' which considered two large groups of disorders: weakness as a constitutional defect (idiots, imbeciles, amentias) and weakness as a secondary phenomenon, i.e. dementia. The latter was divided into primary or acute, 'when it follows some violent strain or shock, physical or mental, which paralyses mental function for a time or for life' (p345)[56]. The latter, in turn, Maudsley considered 'most frequently, but not invariably, secondary to some other form of mental derangement'. Five main causes were identified: 1. attacks of mental disorder which, 'lapse by quick steps of degeneration into terminal dementia', 2. habitual alcoholic excess. 3. frequent fits of established epilepsy, 4. positive damage from physical injury of the brain, and 5. 'failure of nutrition and deterioration of structure from the degeneration changes that condition the brain-decay of old age. The resulting mental decay is known as senile dementia or senile imbecility' (p347).

Maudsley soon realised that to consider the senile dementias as 'secondary' sounded strange, 'although chronic, it is really primary. But old age is virtually the slow natural disease of which a man dies at last when he has no other disease; one need not scruple, therefore, to describe his dotage as secondary. Moreover, there is the unanswerable argument that it is secondary to the feverish disease of life' (pp347-348). But there is also a sadder side to this affair. In the early 1890s, Mrs Maudsley seems to have developed a form of senile dementia which led her devoted husband to give up most of his commitments to look after her. Since by all accounts her life was a rather tranquil one, would Maudsley still have felt able to say that all dementias were, after all, secondary to the 'feverish disease of life'?

Clouston

In 1887, Thomas Clouston classified mental disorders as states of mental depression (psychalgia, such as melancholia), mental exaltation (psychlampsia, such as mania), and mental enfeeblement (dementia, amentia, congenital imbecility, and idiocy). He suggested that there were: 'two great physiological periods of mental enfeeblement, viz. in childhood and old age . . . if the brain development is arrested before birth or in childhood, we have congenital imbecility and idiocy—amentia. Dotage must be reckoned as natural at the end of life. It is not actually the same as senile dementia, but there is no scientific difference' (p267)[57].

Though distinguishing five types of dementia, Clouston suggested that every one was incurable, and that 'the medical profession outside of public institutions has little to do with its treatment or management' (p271). However, he considered secondary dementia (or vesanic for the French) the commonest variety, and tried to identify clinical markers that could predict when a patient with mania or melancholia might develop dementia. 'Senile dementia' was discussed under the 'senile insanities': i.e. on account of their age, a proportion of people develop a chronic and incurable condition which should be called dementia. His views are typical of the period, in that senile dementia starts to be classified as a separate and primary group, but not much is said about its causes or clinical features; the commonest way out of this dilemma was to see it as an exaggeration of physiological senility, or as a form of vesanic dementia.

Crichton Browne

In 1874, Crichton Browne, director of the West Riding Asylum[58], delivered a lecture on dementia whose modern-sounding clinical remarks became influential only amongst early twentieth-century figures such as Shaw Bolton and Mott. He described three cases— one of agitated depression, another of senile mania, and the third of a typical senile dementia; although most clinicians might have grouped them together as instances of 'senile insanity', he considered them different diseases. Senile dementia was a condition in which there was 'a failure of memory, especially as to recent events . . . Long past occurrences, the incidents of youth and boyhood, may readily be recollected' (p601)[59]. He believed this failure to be due not only to 'dullness in perception . . . but also to enfeeblement of the conservative powers themselves'. Delusions and hallucinations were said to be part of the condition, although they may on occasions be 'dilapidated' (p602); emotions were also blunted, and there were marked changes in personality and physical appearance. He differentiated senile from 'apoplectic' dementia and claimed that although vascular changes might be present on occasions, 'senile dementia may occur without any vascular degeneration' (p602).

Sir George Savage
Sir George Savage also divided dementia into two categories: 'In one there is a destruction more or less complete of the mind, which can never be recovered from, and in the other there is a functional arrest, which may pass off . . . at the one end of life there may be inability to develop intellectually . . . amentia; and at the other end destruction of mind may leave the whole intellectual fabric a ruin . . . dementia' (p207)[60].

Earlier, he had proposed the concept of 'partial dementia': 'Young adults, who have given way to excesses, especially when several varieties of excess have been indulged in at the same time, become unable to perform the duties for which they have been educated and fully prepared'. This was illustrated by a decline in performance and symptoms in a case of simple schizophrenia. However, his new category did not thrive. In the fourth edition of the *Nomenclature of Diseases* of the Royal College of Physicians, the dementias were classified under the 'degenerations' (p39)[61] and considered as being of two types: primary and secondary; there were also six varieties, including senile and organic. Savage was one of the advisors on mental diseases to the committee preparing this edition.

Joseph Shaw Bolton
Whilst at the turn of the century most alienists were trying to improve the classification of the dementias in terms of an analysis of their clinical symptoms, Bolton, at Claybury Hospital, Essex started post-mortem studies which he hoped might serve as the basis for a neuropathological classification. He divided his patients into four main groups: insanity without dementia, insanity with dementia, dementia with insanity, and severe dementia. To avoid brain lysis, Bolton stored the corpses soon after death in the cold chamber developed by Mott years earlier. Based on studies of cortical neurons, Bolton offered a classification in 1903 which included amentia, mental confusion, and dementia, and the latter was subdivided into: the 'dementia of worn-out neurones . . . dementia of degenerates who owing to stress have become insane and . . . the dementia of degenerates which is associated with premature vascular degeneration' (p550)[62]. That not all patients' histories fitted into his classification, Bolton explained by the fact that 'patients die at all stages of their mental diseases' (p550).

However, this classification, like others based on one or two aetiological principles, did not last beyond the First World War. The theory of degeneration, which since Morel had provided a crucial explanation for all classifications of dementia, went out of favour, and with it disappeared the local versions of the doctrine, such as that of 'abiotrophy'—sponsored in England by William Gowers[63]. Neurologists also became interested in the dementias, particularly those related to putative vascular changes. Finally, new forms of dementia were described, such as Creutzfeld-Jakob disease[64] and the Von Economo defect states[65], which did not fit into the old groupings. It is not surprising, therefore, that by the 1930s, the most popular classification in England was that propounded by a neurologist, Macdonald Critchley[66]. He gave up the idea of identifying a common aetiological denominator, and simply listed the main groups of dementias: syphilitic, arteriosclerotic, traumatic, due to space-occupying lesions, epileptic, following chronic neurological and psychotic diseases, toxic-infective, and 'essential'— which included Alzheimer's and Pick's disease. When Mayer-Gross (1944) was asked to review this field for the *Journal of Mental Science*, he limited himself to confirming Critchley's classification[67].

OVERVIEW

By the 1860s, the clinical boundaries of dementia had begun to be narrowed down by separating off clinical states such as stupor, the vesanic dementias, melancholic pseudodementia, and most of the cognitive defects relating to brain injury. The end-result was a more or less homogeneous clinical group that contained only senile and arteriosclerotic dementias. The historical forces that guided this process included the development of morbid anatomy[68], the reaffirmation in psychology of emphasis on the intellectual (cognitive) functions[69], and the view that senility was an exaggerated and/or pathological form of ageing[70].

Neuropathological research, of which the work of Alzheimer is a classical example, was based on a 'correlational' paradigm—the nineteenth-century anatomo-clinical model of disease—that changes in tissues or organs were expressed as signs and symptoms[71]. This led to efforts to improve both histological techniques and the clinical definition and measurement of the state of dementia.

The choice of cognitive failure as the hallmark of dementia was determined by many factors: it reflected the clinical facts—observation showed institutionalised patients to have cognitive incompetence, but eliciting subjective experiences was difficult in demented subjects. Intellect was still considered the defining feature of the human species; not only was madness defined in 'intellectualistic' terms, but after the 1860s, the view had become popular that psychosocial incompetence, whether in the mentally ill, the elderly, idiots, or members of non-European races, specifically resulted from intellectual failure. This ideology was related to degeneration theory—the belief that acquired social perversions (such as alcoholism) caused behavioural and physical stigmata which would be passed to later generations in the form of melancholia, mania, and finally dementia[72]. It is no coincidence that the great preoccupation of the British Eugenics movement (founded by Francis Galton, Charles Darwin's cousin and Karl Pearson) was the intellectual betterment of the race[73]. The development of the 'cognitive paradigm' was guided by both clinical and ideological trends.

Cognition, however, proved too broad a function to measure. Those interested in the assessment of severity resorted to memory, the only intellectual function whose measurement had reached adequate development during the 1880s[74]. Thus, deficits in memory became, *de facto*, if not *de jure*, the central feature of the state of dementia. The ensuing cognitive paradigm has served the profession well but may need broadening, particularly in relation to the clinical evaluation of the states of early and advanced dementia. It is hoped that this chapter will have helped to identify those clinical aspects of dementia which were left aside in the process that established the conceptual basis for today's Alzheimer's disease.

Chapter 3

Alzheimer and His Time

P. Hoff

This chapter attempts to give a comprehensive overview of Alzheimer's life, the historical background of his scientific work, and its relationship to the ideas of other distinguished authors of his time. The growth of interest in this topic in recent decades is reflected by an increasing number of publications[1-13].

Biographical background

Alois Alzheimer was born on the 14th of June, 1864, in the Lower Franconian village of Marktbreit am Main, near Würzburg. The house where he was born has only recently been identified and marked with a commemorative plaque. He was the second child in the family, his father being a notary. After studying locally and in Aschaffenburg, another picturesque town in the province, he took his final examinations at the Royal Humanistic Secondary School in 1883 and received a certificate with the commendation, 'exceptional knowledge in the sciences'. He studied medicine in Berlin, Würzburg, and Tübingen; in 1887, he passed his examinations for the degree of doctor of medicine and a year later concluded his final state medical qualification. He wrote his dissertation thesis on the histology of the ceruminous glands[14] (Fig. 1). Alzheimer first worked for the anatomist Albert Kolliker (1817-1905) in Wurzburg, but stayed in this position for only one term. According to his personal records, he spent the following five months accompanying a 'mentally ill lady' on her travels, a common position for junior doctors at this time; his interest in psychiatry seems to have begun after this[15].

From 1888 until 1902, i.e. from his 24th until his 38th year, Alzheimer worked as an assistant medical officer and then from 1895 as a senior medical officer at the Municipal Mental Asylum in Frankfurt am Main under the directorship of Emil Sioli (1852-1922). There, he developed a close personal and professional relationship with Franz Nissl (1860-1919), which resulted in their scientific partnership.

He was a close friend of W Erb who had treated a banker for syphilis and at the end of the treatment, the banker financed a scientific expedition to North Africa on the proviso that he and his wife would accompany the team. They had just arrived in Algeria when the banker had a mental breakdown. Erb contacted Alzheimer,

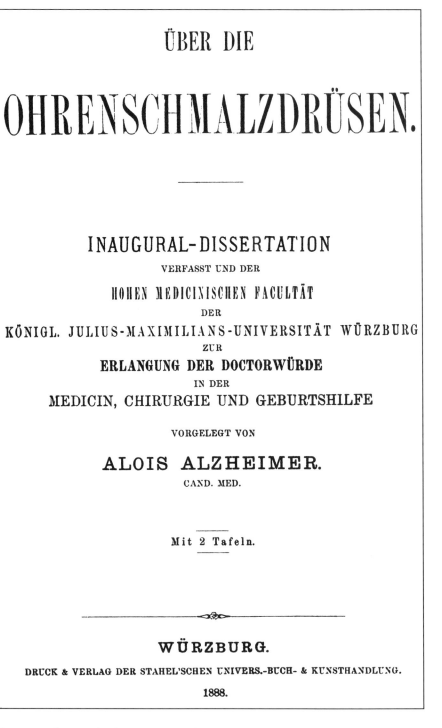

Figure 1 Cover of Alzheimer's Medical Dissertation 'On ceruminal glands', Würzburg, 1888 (ref. 1).

who came to Algeria to bring the patient and his wife back to Germany. When the banker died, Alzheimer married his widow, Cecilia Geisenheimer, in Frankfurt in April 1894, Nissl being witness at the wedding. The couple had three children, a son and two daughters (Fig. 2). One of the daughters married his co-worker in Breslau, Georg Stertz (1878-1959), who later became Professor of Psychiatry in Munich. Alzheimer never overcame his wife's early death in February, 1901.

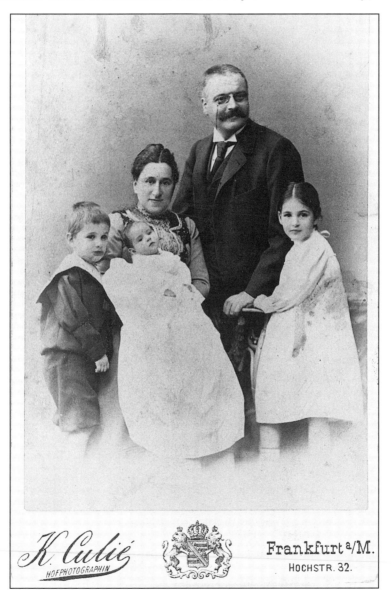

Figure 2 Alzheimer and his family, 1900/1901 (courtesy of Mrs H Köppen, Wessling).

Originally, Alzheimer was apparently not interested in a scientific career, but instead intended to apply for a position as director of an asylum. Emil Kraepelin (1856-1926) must have known this; he had become Professor of Psychiatry in Heidelberg in 1891, and wanted Alzheimer to work together with Nissl in his anatomical laboratory. However, Kraepelin's offer led to a major change in Alzheimer's plans, although he was hesitant about this decision. Kraepelin seemed to be astonished about this hesitation, which is reflected by the slight irony in the following remarks in his memoirs:

'The prospects became better in this field of research, when it became possible that Alzheimer might move to Heidelberg. I had heard by chance some time previously that this excellent research worker was about to apply for the job of director of an asylum. A mutual friend intervened on my behalf and urgently requested him not to make such a step, but to start an academic career. Unfortunately, this advice was not successful at first and it was not until Alzheimer's attempts to become director of an asylum failed that he came to me and I persuaded him to join our group. Before his habilitation in Heidelberg took place, I was appointed to the professorial chair in Munich and Alzheimer came to Munich with me.' (p106)[16].

Nissl, however, stayed in Heidelberg and became Kraepelin's successor—at least for some years: he too was persuaded later by Kraepelin to come to Munich. But unlike Alzheimer, who was to leave his Munich laboratory in order to take over the chair of psychiatry in Breslau, Nissl renounced his professorship in Heidelberg so as to concentrate on scientific work. In 1918, Nissl became head of the department of histopathology at the newly founded *Deutsche Forschungsanstalt für Psychiatrie* in Munich. These years around the end of World War I were unfortunate, though, both for the field of psychiatric research and for Kraepelin personally: in his essay, *Lebensschicksale deutscher Forscher*[17] he expressed his deep concern about the fact that three important representatives of histopathology of the CNS in Germany had died within only five years: Alois Alzheimer in 1915, Korbinian Brodmann in 1918, and Franz Nissl in 1919.

By the time Alzheimer arrived in Heidelberg from Frankfurt in 1903, Kraepelin had become disillusioned with the Ministry of the Interior; apparently influenced by the head of the Illenau Asylum, it had not kept its promise of extending his clinical facilities at the University Clinic. This had been founded in 1878, but by Kraepelin's time it was severely overcrowded, with patients having to be bedded down in the corridors or straw mattresses. Kraepelin was offered the Munich chair in June 1903, but delayed acceptance to give the Ministry yet another chance. However, still nothing happened and he left for Munich in October, Alzheimer moving with him[16].

From 1903 to 1912, his years in Munich, Alzheimer became a well loved figure to students from all over the world. He would spend hours with each one, explaining things as they shared a microscope, always with a cigar which would be put down as he commenced his explanations, and it is said that at the end of the day there would always be a cigar stump at every student's bench by the micro-scope. He remained as Kraepelin's co-worker; since the university was completing a new building for the Psychiatric Clinic at the Nussbaumstrasse near the centre of the city, both Kraepelin and Alzheimer had the opportunity to discuss and influence the final planning. The official opening ceremony was held on November 4th, 1904 (Fig. 3). In the same year, Alzheimer was promoted to University Lecturer with his habilitation thesis 'Histological studies on the differential diagnoses of general paresis'[18] (Fig. 4). Alzheimer's anatomical laboratory was to become one of the important centres of histopathological research.

However, Alzheimer did not have the opportunity to concentrate fully on his scientific projects while working in Munich. After Robert Gaupp had left the Munich hospital to take over the chair of psy-chiatry at the university of Tübingen in 1906, Kraepelin wondered who would be most competent as Gaupp's successor and his own deputy:

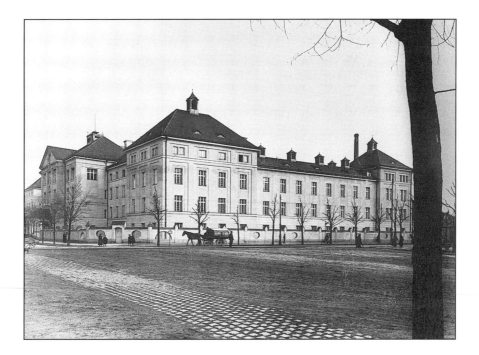

Figure 3   The 'Royal Psychiatric Hospital' of the University of Munich, about 1904.

'The choice of a suitable successor caused me considerable problems. I knew no person more suitable than my faithful colleague Alzheimer. . . . I asked him to accept the post of Senior Assistant at least for the time being. This meant a great sacrifice on his part, as he would have to give up the absolute freedom of

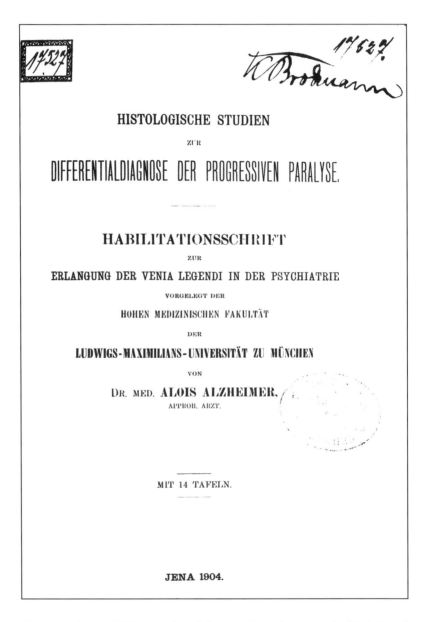

Figure 4 Cover of Alzheimer's habilitation thesis from 1904 (ref. 24) signed 'K. Brodmann' (courtesy of Max-Planck-Institute of Psychiatry, Munich).

his scientific work and he took such commitments seriously. He agreed reluctantly under the condition that he could resign after a reasonable period of time.'[16] (p148).

Since Kraepelin used to leave Munich as soon as the university term was over—he often spent several weeks at his house at Pallanza on Lago Maggiore, working on his textbook—Alzheimer was fully responsible not only for the clinical work, but also for all issues of hospital organisation and education during these months. He held the post of Senior Assistant for three years, i.e. up to 1909, when it was taken over by Ernst Rüdin. 'Once again Alzheimer was free to continue his large-scale scientific studies.'[16] (p149).

In 1912, Alois Alzheimer was appointed ordinary professor and director of the psychiatric hospital in Breslau (Figs. 5 and 6). Kraepelin strongly suspected that 'the very best he (i.e. Alzheimer) had to offer our science would be lost in such a position. Nevertheless, the difficulties and scattered activities in his new job seemed to satisfy him. Unfortunately, he fell ill with an infectious tonsillitis accompanied by nephritis and arthritis and took a long time to recover. I saw him again at the German Psychiatrist Meeting in Breslau in 1913. Although he appeared to be robust, he was depressed and despondent; he was worried by the gloomy future. It was our last meeting. Alzheimer tried to fulfil his responsibilities and duties to the utmost. In the increasingly difficult conditions during the war, he was forced to take on one new assignment after the other. His health deteriorated noticeably and finally this excellent man and scientist succumbed to uraemia without having solved the great problem and without having shown us the pathological anatomy of mental disorders, although he was better qualified than anyone else.'[16] (p149). Alois Alzheimer died of rheumatic endocarditis in Breslau on December 19, 1915, only 51 years of age.

The development of Alzheimer's scientific ideas

Historical views on well-known representatives of different psychiatric schools sometimes suffer from a tendency to simplify biographical as well as theoretical aspects of their stories. Emil Kraepelin, whose life and work are closely related to Alzheimer's, is regarded as a highly influential German psychiatrist of the beginning of this century, holding the Chair of Psychiatry at the University of Munich, who was predominantly interested in nosological issues and introduced the dichotomy of endogenous psychoses—'dementia praecox' versus 'manic-depressive insanity'. All these facts are true, but they represent only a part of what deserves to be mentioned if a balanced judgement is to be reached on Kraepelin and 'his' psychiatry.

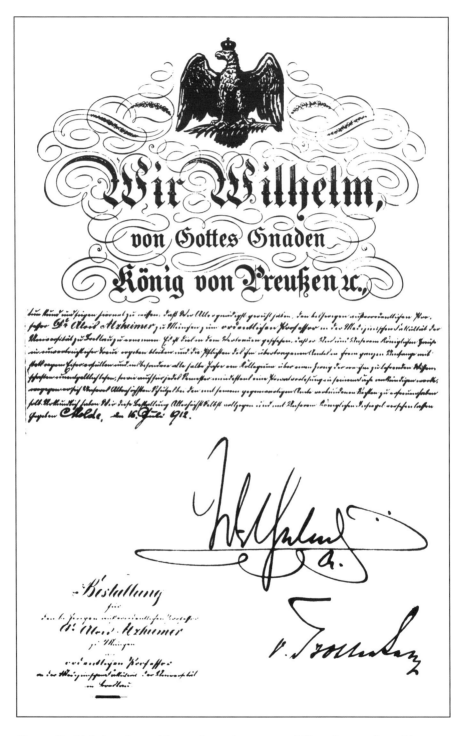

Figure 5   *Alzheimer's certificate of appointment as full professor of psychiatry at the University of Breslau, signed by Wilhelm II, King of Prussia, dated July 16, 1912.*

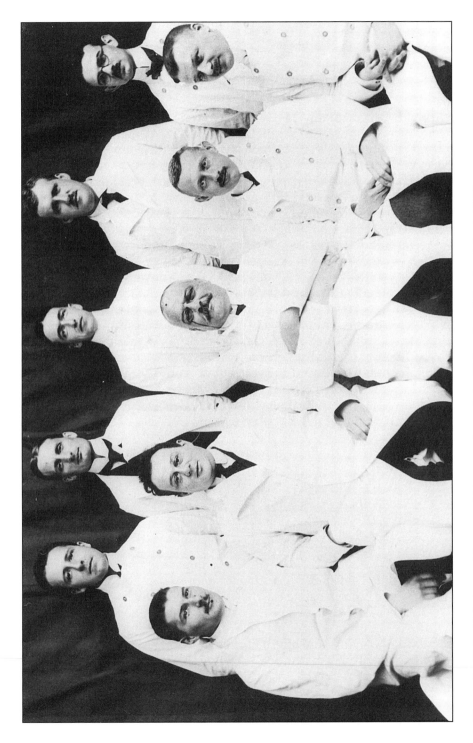

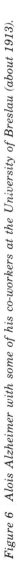

Figure 6   Alois Alzheimer with some of his co-workers at the University of Breslau (about 1913).

A second example is Alzheimer himself. Through greatly increased research activities in the field of dementia, his name is now known world-wide as the 'discoverer' of a 'presenile' type of dementia which was later named after him. But little is known about the man himself and—astonishingly enough—not much more about his widespread scientific work, which was by no means limited to studies of dementing processes, nor even to histopathological research in general. The development of his work cannot be understood without taking into account the complex background of eighteenth- and nineteenth-century scientific theory and philosophy[19,20]. In his theoretical paper on 'The diagnostic difficulties in psychiatry' of 1910, Alzheimer specified what he saw as the crucial issues in conceptualising psychiatric illness: 'The most urgent task of any medical science is the collection of single cases in the form of diseases, which within certain boundaries are defined by their aetiology and their relevant features concerning clinical phenomenology and outcome.'[21] Like this first sentence, the rest of the text shows many similarities with Kraepelin's thinking, even down to the level of single words, and this similarity is by no means accidental.

The most important teachers who influenced Alzheimer when he started working in clinical psychiatry in 1888 were Emil Sioli and Franz Nissl. Sioli (1852-1922) was director of the mental hospital of Frankfurt am Main. Immediately after taking over this position in 1888, he had introduced the concept of 'non-restraint'[22] into the hospital, which considerably improved both the therapeutic atmosphere and the reputation of the institution as a progressive one. Alzheimer praised Sioli's initiatives in his 1913 essay 'Twenty-five Years of Psychiatry'[23].

In Frankfurt, Alzheimer also met the anatomist and pathologist Carl Weigert (1845-1904), who had been the director of the Senckenberg Institute there since 1884. Ludwig Edinger (1855-1918), who later became Professor of Neurology, also worked at the same institute. The work of Weigert and Edinger would naturally have attracted Alzheimer, who had already shown his interest in anatomy and histology as a medical student in Würzburg, but the encounter with Franz Nissl was probably the most important one. A short time before, Nissl had developed a method to improve the staining of nerve cells and their inner structures (Nissl-Farbung), which soon proved a powerful research tool in neuroanatomy, being adopted in many laboratories in different countries. Again, it was Sioli who early on recognised his talents and offered him a position as senior physician. Nissl, up to then living in Munich, accepted this in 1889, one year after Alzheimer had come to the hospital; a close professional relationship developed between Alzheimer and Nissl, who was four years older. Together, they introduced progressive developments into the methods and content of the histopathology of the CNS, though compared to Nissl, Alzheimer laid more emphasis on gathering clinical experience.

During the 14 years he spent at the Frankfurt hospital, Alzheimer published 20 papers which mainly but not exclusively dealt with inflammatory and vascular brain diseases through histological and histochemical methods[24-43] (Fig. 7). Here, Alzheimer concentrated on mental disorders with clear organic causes, as shown by such papers as 'Arteriosclerotic brain atrophy'[26] or 'A case of luetic meningomyelitis and -encephalitis'[33]. Walter Spielmeyer[44] describes this as the first half of Alzheimer's life-work, which went as far as the habilitation thesis, 'Histological studies on the differential diagnosis of general paresis' of 1904[18]. In the second phase from 1904 until 1915, Alzheimer's interest progressively shifted to what is referred to as 'endogenous' psychoses in ICD-9, but no

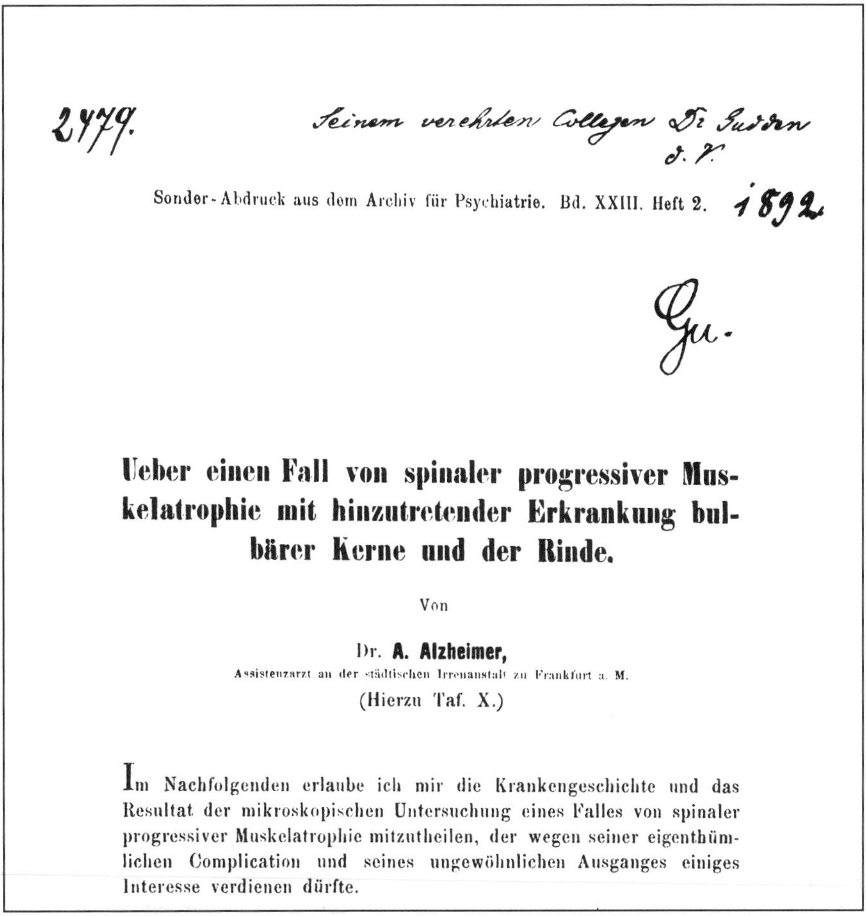

2479.

Seinem verehrten Collegen Dr Gudden
d. V.

Sonder-Abdruck aus dem Archiv für Psychiatrie. Bd. XXIII. Heft 2.   1892.

Gu.

Ueber einen Fall von spinaler progressiver Muskelatrophie mit hinzutretender Erkrankung bulbärer Kerne und der Rinde.

Von

Dr. A. Alzheimer,
Assistenzarzt an der städtischen Irrenanstalt zu Frankfurt a. M.

(Hierzu Taf. X.)

Im Nachfolgenden erlaube ich mir die Krankengeschichte und das Resultat der mikroskopischen Untersuchung eines Falles von spinaler progressiver Muskelatrophie mitzutheilen, der wegen seiner eigenthümlichen Complication und seines ungewöhnlichen Ausganges einiges Interesse verdienen dürfte.

Figure 7   Alzheimer's study on progressive spinal muscular atrophy (1892) (ref. 2), with handwritten dedication to 'his honourable colleague Dr Gudden', whose initials ('Gu') are written below.

longer in ICD-10. As a clinician, he clearly felt that he had to accept the challenge of applying his histopathological methods to patients with dementia praecox and manic-depressive insanity. However, already during his time in Frankfurt, Alzheimer had published on the pathological anatomy of chronic mental disorders[41], thereby indicating the direction his research was going to take after 1904. Furthermore, there are many examples of his constant interest in issues beyond histopathology, during his 27 years of practice in clinical psychiatry (*vide infra*).

Since forensic psychiatry was not yet regarded as a separate and specialised field at that time, every clinician was familiar with it, and many authors like Alzheimer, Bonhoeffer, and Kraepelin—generally known for quite different topics—produced work on forensic topics. At the age of 24, Kraepelin had published an important and provoking study on 'The abolition of the degree of punishment' (*Die Abschaffung des Strafmasses*)[45], calling in question elements of the penal code of that time. Alzheimer, however, though sharing an interest in the subject, preferred to combine the detailed description of clinical cases with theoretical considerations. For example, in 1896 he published a case report on a fetishist, 'teacher and former candidate of theology O.', who had been charged several times with fraud and larceny[30]. A previous psychiatric expert, Dr Kurella, senior physician at the mental hospital in Brieg/Silesia, had judged this person to be simulating and mentally undisturbed, a shrewd defrauder, and fully reponsible according to the penal code. In opposition to this, Alzheimer argued that the accused was suffering from a severe psychological disorder which had grown worse over time, restricting his degree of freedom and excluding his penal responsibility.

The fact that forensic issues were felt then to be of great importance was not only for practical reasons: it was also related to the politically and scientifically influential concept of 'degeneration'. These ideas were promoted by Cesare Lombroso's Italian School of Criminology[46], which closely connected criminal behaviour with onto- and phylogenetic retardation. Alzheimer's emphasis on degeneration (in a non-anatomical sense) corresponded with the views of the psychiatrist Paul-Julius Möbius, who had supported the distinction between 'exogenous' and 'endogenous' mental disorders in German-speaking psychiatry[47,48]. In clinical psychopathology, H Schule, R v Krafft-Ebing, and two French authors, BA Morel and JJ-V Magnan were also influential supporters of a degenerationist view, although their basic theoretical orientation was very different, Morel being strongly influenced by Christian moral philosophy and Magnan by the empirical methodology of natural sciences[46-48,49-51]. Alzheimer's position in this matter was a differentiated one: on the one hand, he rejected the crude and purely speculative statement that the existence of a mental disorder as such proved the degenerate state of the patient. On the other, he defended the concept of 'inherited degenerative mental disorders', regarding his forensic patient O as an excellent example of this; the title of his case report, 'A born criminal'[30], refers to the Lombrosian tradition. However, Alzheimer's critical and clinically orientated position is indicated by the fact that he put the term 'born criminal' in quotation marks. Furthermore, he added ironically that in spite of the 'exceptionally eager research' of Lombroso and his pupils, nobody had succeeded in 'defining a cluster of stigmata of degeneration separating the criminal from the insane.'[30] From his own degenerationist point of view, Alzheimer would probably have considered it more appropriate to call his forensic patient a 'born fetishist', rather than a 'born criminal'.

He also published studies and case reports on the differential diagnosis of mental deficiency as it occurs in cases of tuberous sclerosis or amaurotic family idiocy, and criticised the practice of treating most of the severely mentally retarded in non-medical institutions, since this constituted an obstacle to psychiatric education and research[52]. In most of his papers, Alzheimer took the opportunity to emphasise the relevance of empirically based clinical concepts, especially when applying terms like 'dementia', which have a long and, even for nineteenth-century authors, puzzling conceptual history.[19] Describing the best way out of this terminological vagueness, Alzheimer used almost the same words as Kraepelin in the fifth edition (1896) of his textbook: 'Symptomatological description has been replaced by a clinical one.'[52]

In 1907, Alzheimer considered the problem of 'Indications for induced abortion in mentally ill women'[53], which had become controversial after Jolly had proposed very broad criteria at a meeting in Hamburg in 1901. Alzheimer discussed several hypotheses on the aetiology and nosology of gestational psychosis, but unlike Jolly, did not accept manic-depressive insanity as an indication for induced abortion. Since the course of illness in dementia praecox was said not to be significantly influenced by pregnancy, this disease too was not a sufficient indication. Alzheimer rejected any simplifying social Darwinism, which postulated that the process of degeneration is necessarily intensified in the offspring of mentally ill patients. He argued that empirical support was lacking for such a strong and pessimistic hypothesis, and that there might equally be a kind of 'regenerating tendency'. His narrow indications for induced abortion, compared with Jolly's, were substantiated mainly by clinical arguments.

Alzheimer also carried out several investigations into epilepsy[35,39,54-56]. These aimed at a more exact symptomatological and nosological definition of the term 'epilepsy', and dealt particularly with the development of histopathological criteria for the differential diagnosis between 'genuine' epilepsy and symptomatic convulsive disorder.

Furthermore, his position at the Munich hospital as well as probably the preparations for taking over the chair in Breslau stimulated his interest in questions of mental health policy. Here again, there was a parallel between him and Kraepelin, the latter being one of the most active—and polemical—promoters of the social

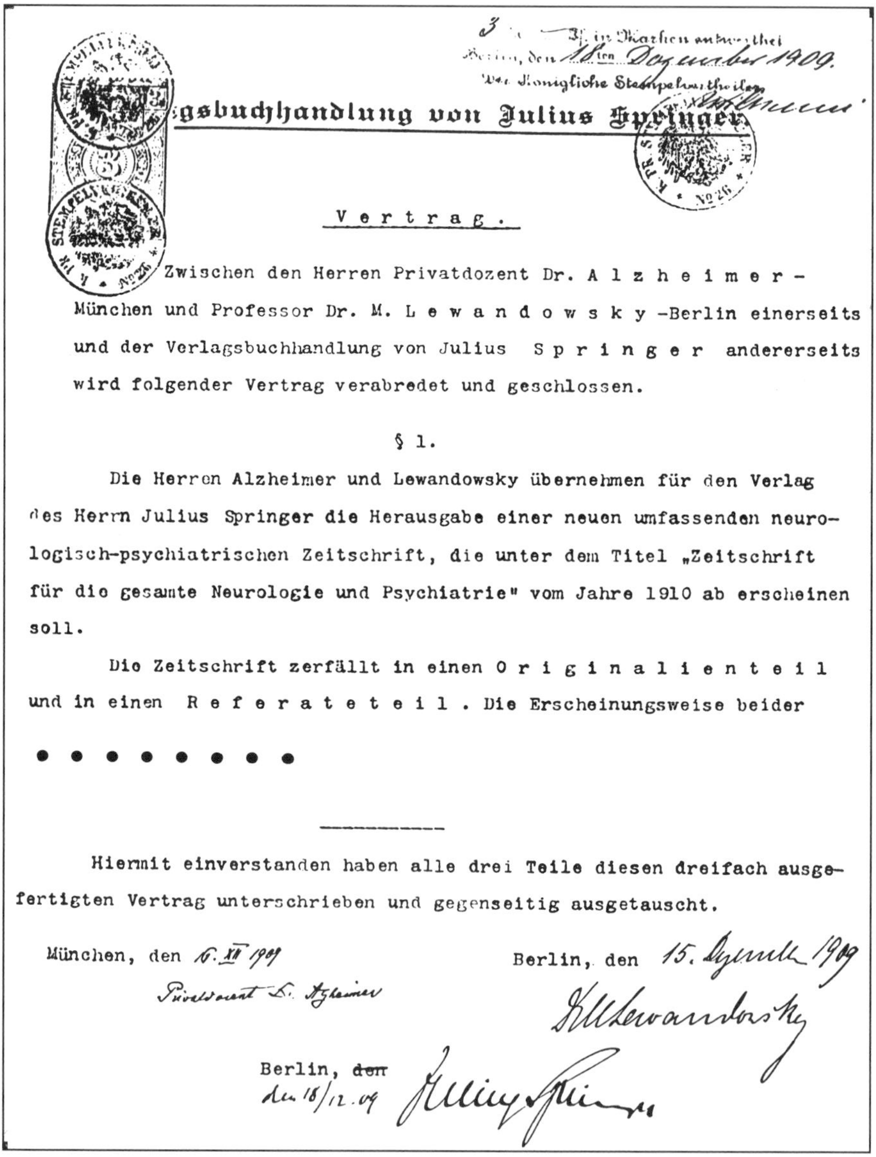

...gsbuchhandlung von Julius Springer

Vertrag.

Zwischen den Herren Privatdozent Dr. Alzheimer-München und Professor Dr. M. Lewandowsky-Berlin einerseits und der Verlagsbuchhandlung von Julius Springer andererseits wird folgender Vertrag verabredet und geschlossen.

§ 1.

Die Herren Alzheimer und Lewandowsky übernehmen für den Verlag des Herrn Julius Springer die Herausgabe einer neuen umfassenden neurologisch-psychiatrischen Zeitschrift, die unter dem Titel „Zeitschrift für die gesamte Neurologie und Psychiatrie" vom Jahre 1910 ab erscheinen soll.

Die Zeitschrift zerfällt in einen Originalienteil und in einen Referateteil. Die Erscheinungsweise beider

• • • • • • • •

Hiermit einverstanden haben alle drei Teile diesen dreifach ausgefertigten Vertrag unterschrieben und gegenseitig ausgetauscht.

München, den 16. XII 1909 — Privatdozent Dr. Alzheimer

Berlin, den 15. Dezember 1909 — M Lewandowsky

Berlin, ~~den~~ den 18/12.09 — Julius Springer

Figure 8 Contract between Springer-Verlag, A Alzheimer and M Lewandowsky on the edition of the 'Journal for the entire neurology and psychiatry' (Zeitschrift für die gesamte Neurologie und Psychiatrie), *December 1909 (courtesy of Springer-Verlag, Heidelberg).*

and political relevance of psychiatric theories, such as the influence of alcoholism. In 1911, Alzheimer commented on plans to found a department of psychiatry in the *Reichsgesundheitsamt*[57], which had been proposed by the psychiatrist R Sommer at the International Congress of Mental Health Care in Berlin, the previous autumn. Alzheimer stressed the necessity of what would now be called psychiatric epidemiology, referring to long-standing controversies about the reasons for the steadily growing number of chronic patients in mental hospitals. His catalogue of the functions which should be carried out by such an institute has many similarities to Kraepelin's much more elaborated paper of 1916, which embodied his plans for a 'German Research Institute of Psychiatry'.[58]

From 1909 until his death, Alzheimer was the editor of the psychiatric section of the *Zeitschrift für die gesamte Neurologie und Psychiatrie*, whilst Lewandowsky was responsible for the neurological part (Fig. 8). This evidence of the wide range of Alzheimer's scientific work provides the background to two issues, which are the most important from a present-day point of view. The first is his description of 'presenile dementia' and the second his strict orientation on Kraepelinian nosology or, in a more general sense, on a Kraepelinian way of defining psychiatry as a medical science.

The history of 'Alzheimer's Disease'
In November 1901, Alzheimer, still working in Frankfurt, examined a 51 year-old woman (AD), who had been admitted to the psychiatric hospital. She presented with a distinct decrease in perceptivity and memory, as well as aphasia, lack of orientation, unpredictable behaviour, paranoid ideas, auditory hallucinations, and marked psychosocial incompetence. After her death in April 1906, Alzheimer gave a report on the case at a conference of psychiatrists in Tübingen on November 3rd, (Fig. 9). The title of his lecture was 'On a peculiar disease process of the cerebral cortex' ('*Über eine eigenartige Erkrankung der Hirnrinde*')[59]. In 1910 Gaetano Perusini, Alzheimer's co-worker in Munich, published a paper on 'Clinically and histologically peculiar mental disorders of old age'.[60] The first of his four cases is probably identical with Alzheimer's case of 'AD'[3,61].

Alzheimer's personal impression of the relevance of what he had just described is of interest:

'All things considered, we are obviously concerned here with a peculiar disease process. Such processes have been established in great numbers in recent years. This finding will necessarily induce us not to be content with laboriously forcing any clinically uncertain case into one of our well-known nosological categories. Doubtless, there are many more mental disorders than are listed in our textbooks; in some of these cases, histological analysis will

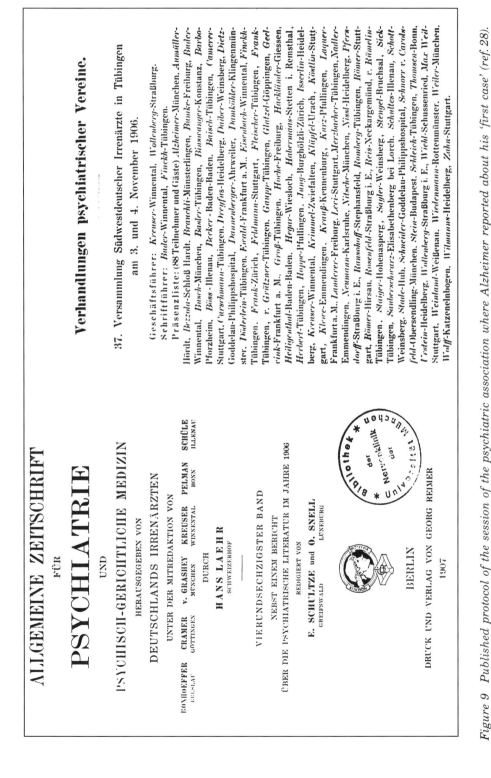

Figure 9   Published protocol of the session of the psychiatric association where Alzheimer reported about his 'first case' (ref. 28).

allow the peculiarity of the case to be identified later. Then, we will gradually reach the point where we will separate single diseases clinically from the large nosological groups of our textbooks and define these large groups clinically in a more precise way.'[59]

Neither Alzheimer himself nor his close co-workers seem to have been fully aware at this early stage that he had 'discovered' an entirely new disease. But following Kraepelin's influential suggestion, this 'presenile dementia' with a diffuse atrophy of the entire brain, but especially of the cortex, together with the various changes in the inner structure of the neurons, was later called 'Alzheimer's disease' or 'Morbus Alzheimer'. In his comprehensive study of 1911, Alzheimer seems surprised when he states that 'Kraepelin in the eighth edition of his textbook on psychiatry has already given a short summary of these diseases and called them Alzheimer's disease.'[62] After a review of the contemporary literature (Bonfiglio, Fischer, Hübner, Myake, Perusini, Pick, Redlich, Sarteschi, Simchowicz), he discussed whether or not the cases he had regarded as peculiar should be separated clinically or histologically from senile dementia.

In recent years, there has been much speculation as to why Kraepelin so readily accepted that Alzheimer's clinical and histopathological description should constitute a new and distinct disease entity. Were there mainly scientific reasons, as proposed by Beach[2], or was it that the strongest motive came from Kraepelin's desire to add prestige to his Munich laboratory, either in order to demonstrate the superiority of his 'school' over psychoanalytic concepts or — more likely — over the competing group in Prague headed by Arnold Pick.[1,63]

Oskar Fischer, one of Pick's co-workers, had in fact published interesting histopathological findings on senile dementia in 1907[64]. However, from an historical point of view, none of these hypotheses about Kraepelin's motives for coining the term 'Alzheimer's disease' so quickly can be regarded as definitely proven.[61]

Alzheimer & Kraepelin

Although the influence of Nissl on Alzheimer is clear so far as histopathology is concerned, that of Kraepelinian thought on his basic clinical concepts is equally so. After following Kraepelin to Munich in 1903, Alzheimer laid more emphasis on the histopathology of dementia praecox and manic-depressive illness, later defined as the two large groups of 'endogenous' psychoses. However, there were considerable differences between the meaning of this term for Alzheimer and, for example, for Kurt Schneider. Six of Alzheimer's publications deal directly with these questions[32,41,65-68]. His lengthy study from 1912[66] still focused on general paresis, whereas his 1913 paper commented on the key topic of, 'The understanding of the pathological-anatomical process underlying dementia praecox'[67].

Being a clear-cut 'Kraepelinian' himself, Alzheimer was forced to take Bleuler's position into account: he noted that 'since Bleuler's interesting monograph, there is much discussion on the psychopathology of schizophrenia'. However, there is an unmistakably disappointed undertone when he called the available data on histopathology 'rather insufficient', i.e. not convincing enough to support Bleuler's hypotheses[67]. He reported here on 55 cases of dementia praecox, calling the impairment of glial and neuronal elements of the cerebral cortex 'rather considerable'. It might even be possible, he suggested, to use his findings for the differential diagnosis between dementia praecox and mixed states of manic-depressive illness 'in single cases', though it would be too early to assume the clinical picture of dementia praecox from the localisation of the histopathological lesion[67].

Alzheimer rated histopathological methods highly, and was always optimistic that they would produce new and clinically relevant evidence. These concepts and hopes did not suffer the same fate as the speculative theories of, for example, Theodor Meynert[69] in Vienna, which were often referred to in the literature (e.g. by Kraepelin) as 'brain mythology'. Nor did Alzheimer have naive illusions: when the well-known clinician and neuropathologist Otto Binswanger spoke highly of histopathological studies at a meeting of the Psychiatric Association in 1906, Alzheimer himself warned that not too much should be expected from his efforts to get closer to the anatomical basis of the functional psychoses[65].

In his reviews of the literature, as for example in his 1912 paper, Alzheimer took critical arguments into account:

'The value of pathological anatomy for the further development of clinical psychiatry is rated very differently nowadays. In his book on Cesare Lombroso, Kurella, for example, expresses the opinion that pathological anatomy of psychoses has not produced many positive results, not even in the hands of virtuosi in the art of staining cerebral fibres. Ziehen argues that despite all naive illusions, the pathological-anatomical point of view has failed and further will continue to fail with respect to many psychoses. . . . Kraepelin, however, has considered anatomical findings when describing very different mental disorders. And it cannot be denied that as a result, the essence of some mental disorders has become more understandable, which constitutes a major improvement of clinical psychiatry.'[66]

Bresler[70] concluded that Alzheimer's studies threw light not only on general paresis, senile dementia, arteriosclerosis, and some forms of cerebral luetic infection, but even on the 'other psychoses', by which he meant dementia praecox and manic-depressive insanity. A footnote recorded that Alzheimer had been awarded the Möbius-Prize in recognition of his work on the histopathology of psychotic states.

During his time in Munich, Alzheimer was inevitably involved in the lively scientific discussion that was going on there about the basic questions of psychiatric nosology. In this context, however, the inner structure of Kraepelin's clinic is relevant: major scientific efforts were being made to describe exactly the symptomatology and the clinical course of as many psychotic patients as possible, in order to generate a valid, reliable, and prognostically orientated nosology. Kraepelin's 'leading idea' ('*Leitidee*', as Karl Jaspers put it) was always to 'detect'—not to 'construct'—disease entities which seemed 'natural'. These should be found strictly by empirical means, applying only the amount of theoretical assumption which was absolutely necessary: in philosophical terms, Kraepelin was a 'realist'[71,72].

The influence of the psychologist and philosopher Wilhelm Wundt (1832-1920) on the development of Kraepelin's—and in turn, Alzheimer's—basic ideas about psychiatry and science

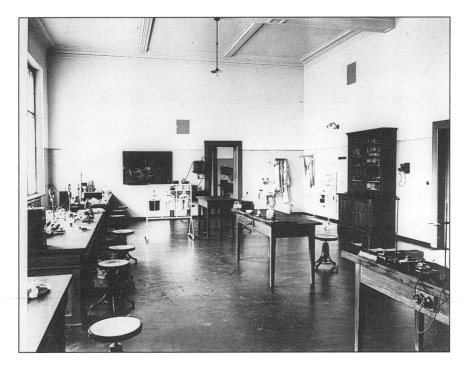

Figure 10   Alzheimer's 'Anatomical Laboratory' in Munich, about 1906.

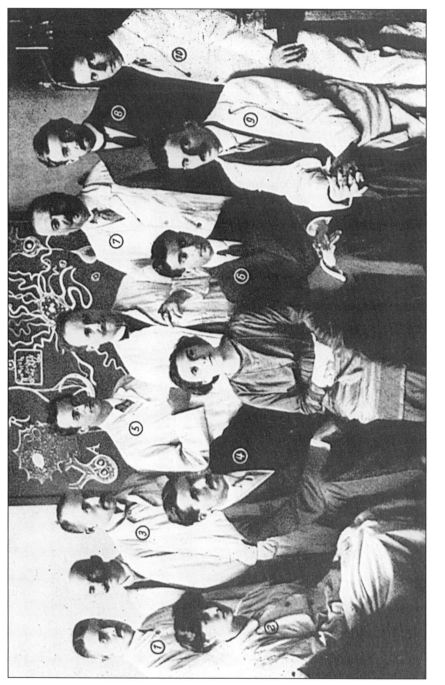

Figure 11 Alzheimer and some of his co-workers in the 'Anatomical Laboratory' in Munich, about 1906; Lotmar 1, Mrs Grombach 2, Rosenthal 3, Cerletti 4, Allers (?) 5, Bonfiglio 6, Alzheimer 7, Achucarro (?) 8, Perusini (?) 9, Lewy 10.

in general can hardly be overestimated. In 1879, Wundt had opened in Leipzig the first institute for experimental psychology and on the basis of psychophysical parallelism, advanced the systematic use of experiments to investigate mental processes, rejecting a purely introspective methodology. Alzheimer's plans to combine clinical psychopathology and histopathology on the theoretical basis of Kraepelin's nosology matched very well Kraepelin's own ideas on how research should be planned and carried out in psychiatry. Kraepelin had continued to discuss these ever since his speech on the occasion of his appointment as Professor of Psychiatry at the Baltic university in Dorpat, published in 1887[73,74].

Apart from these theoretical considerations, what were the practical conditions of Alzheimer's work in Munich? In the earlier years, he was not paid for his work by the university. Alzheimer was able to afford this, due to his wife's large fortune, but a characteristic light is thrown on Kraepelin's personality and on his devotion to psychiatric research in the way he commented on Alzheimer's situation:

'Alzheimer started work in the clinic without being paid, as I had no position for him and he wanted to be able to spend his time as he wished. In order to integrate him into the clinic, I created the class of scientific assistants. This consisted of researchers, who were free to use the scientific facilities and equipment.'[16] (p118).

Appreciating the significance of Alzheimer's ideas for his own understanding of scientific psychiatry, Kraepelin provided him with considerable extra space for his Anatomical Laboratory, situated on the hospital's third floor (Fig. 10). Both the staff and technical equipment of this department were the reasons for its rapidly growing reputation as one of the leading research facilities for the histopathology of the central nervous system. Amongst other co-workers and pupils were G Perusini, F Bonfiglio and UC Cerletti (Italy), HG Creutzfeldt and A Jakob (Germany), and F Lotmar (Switzerland) (Fig. 11). F Nissl joined the group only in 1918, shortly after it had become part of the newly founded German Research Institute, which was situated within the psychiatric hospital at the Nussbaumstrasse in its early years.

Alzheimer therefore had an influential position in the crucial discussions about basic psychiatric topics at the beginning of this century. He often stated that psychiatric research had to be orientated towards clinical questions; as he put it in his habilitation thesis: 'The entire study shall demonstrate that histopathology is a useful auxiliary science for psychiatry.'[18]

The basic philosophical assumptions applied by Kraepelin, especially the 'realistic' approach (in a philosophical sense), were fully accepted by Alzheimer, with a rejection of what was believed to be 'pure speculation'. He regarded Sioli and Kraepelin as his most important clinical teachers, but in contrast to Kraepelin's harsh attacks, Alzheimer's critique of psychoanalysis, for instance, lacked an ironic or polemical undertone. For nosology, Kraepelin's concept was the fundamental framework which he tried to complement and stabilise by empirical, and especially histopathological data.

Alzheimer shared Kraepelin's steadily changing nosological system, throughout the several editions of his textbook, as well as, most importantly, accepting his basic concept of disease entities. This can be demonstrated by Alzheimer's clear position in the controversy between Kraepelin and AE Hoche (1865-1943), which was to become one of the main topics in academic psychiatry after the turn of the century. Here, two publications throw some light on Alzheimer's arguments: the first was his study on diagnostic difficulties in psychiatry[21], and the second his talk at the annual meeting of the German Psychiatric Association at Kiel in 1912[75], the year he moved from Munich to Breslau. Both texts are 'Kraepelinian' through and through, but the longer and more elaborated paper of 1910 represents a critical theoretical reflection on the main topics of psychiatric nosology, whereas the short 1912 paper includes a very lively protocol of the discussion about the relevance of 'symptom complexes' in psychiatry, especially with regard to manic-depressive insanity. Hoche and Alzheimer read papers on this occasion, while Stransky, Kraepelin, Cramer, Siemerling, Weygandt, Meyer, and Cimbal are mentioned as discussants.

The 1910 paper was the very first article to appear in the newly founded *Journal for the entire field of Neurology and Psychiatry*, which demonstrates the importance this topic had for Alzheimer. He dealt with the popular 'anti-Kraepelinian' argument that all efforts to confirm empirically the existence of distinct and 'natural' disease entities had failed, or at least provided psychiatrists with unsatisfyingly 'blurred borders'. Hoche had criticised Kraepelin's position as premature and too speculative. He argued[76,77] that this was not just due to a deplorable lack of methodology, but was the necessary result of a severe conceptual error: to look for natural disease entities was comparable with an uncritical 'chasing after phantoms'. In Hoche's view, Kraepelin's constantly changing nosological system proved the clinical and theoretical unfruitfulness of his basic concept. Hoche demanded a 'syndrome doctrine' in which the syndromes or 'symptom complexes' represent 'second rank units' between the single clinical symptoms and the at least unrecognisable, if even existing 'diseases'.

Alzheimer had too much clinical experience to neglect the difficulties involved in the empirical validation of Kraepelin's nosology, which became evident in the numerous changes that occurred in the classification of paranoid states, for example.

But in his, and of course in Kraepelin's view, these problems
originated in fairly severe methodological, but not fundamental
obstacles to psychiatric research. Thus, the essential problem was
localised not at the theoretical, epistemological level, as Hoche had
argued, but merely at the technical one. Both Kraepelin and
Alzheimer took an optimistic view of the future possibilities for
psychiatric research, and neither gave up this position later on. As
for many other psychiatrists of that time, it was the promising
and paradigmatic example of general paresis, which stimulated
Alzheimer's optimism:

'Twenty years ago, general paresis was not an aetiologically
homogeneous disease. . . . Even outstanding psychiatrists denied
the hypothesis that a syphilitic infection was the necessary
condition. . . . Arteriosclerotic, luetic, alcoholic psychoses could
not be separated. Cases that were cured, got better, or remained
unchanged were mixed together. Today . . . we know that lues
is the only ground on which general paresis can grow. The
prognosis has been clarified; science knows prophylactic methods,
and therapeutic measures can be thought of.'[21].

If Kraepelin's writings on psychiatric nosology are compared with
Alzheimer's, it is Alzheimer who seems more secure and more
convinced. Doubtful remarks are rarely found in his texts, whereas
Kraepelin often mentioned the preliminary status of his nosological
system, which he believed had to be kept open for new clinical
evidence.[78] This does not mean that Kraepelin abandoned his basic
position about the existence and scientific recognisability of natural
disease units. His programmatic studies published between 1918
and 1920 reveal no fundamental differences from his earlier
publications, but he does provide critical reflections on his own
nosology, taking new concepts into account, e.g. Birnbaum's
differentiation between pathogenetic and pathoplastic factors in
psychotic illness[79]. It would be a misunderstanding of Kraepelin's
intentions, therefore, to think that he completely accepted Hoche's
position towards the end of his career. However, such a misunderstanding can easily arise if the following passage is read in
isolation, thus missing its complex connection with the development
of Kraepelin's thinking as a whole:

'We shall have to get accustomed to the idea that the symptoms
we have used up to the present time are not powerful enough to
make possible a reliable distinction between manic-depressive
insanity and schizophrenia. There are overlappings in this field,
which are based on the fact that symptoms are derived from given
preconditions.'[80]

According to this somewhat cryptic formulation, distinct disease processes (*Krankheitsvorgänge*) are still the relevant framework of psychiatric nosology. However, they do not directly create the clinical symptomatology, but are modulated by inborn, preformed psychobiological reaction types. Therefore, symptoms can be nothing more than indicators for, and not proof of the existence of a specific disease — a concept which recalls Karl Bonhoeffer's hypothesis that psychopathological syndromes are 'nosologically non-specific'. This most interesting development in Kraepelin's thinking beyond the eighth edition of his textbook (1909-1915) has been analysed elsewhere[72].

Although, due to his early death in 1915, Alzheimer could not take part in this particular discussion, his acceptance of all the basic Kraepelinian assumptions is evident. In his essay of 1910[21], he apodictically separates 'organic' or 'exogenous' from 'endogenous' or 'functional' psychoses, thus using the terms in a partly, if not completely different sense from today and causing misunderstanding in the literature. Even more emphatically than Kraepelin himself, Alzheimer did not restrict the first, 'exogenous' group to general paresis, but also included schizophrenia, due to his assumption that dementia praecox shows a 'pronounced tendency to end in states of imbecility and due to histological findings'. Manic-depressive illness, however, is in Alzheimer's sense a 'functional' 'endogenous' psychosis; paranoia, hysteria, 'degenerative insanity' (*Entartungsirresein*) and paranoid querulancy were also classified as 'functional'. All mental disorders of this group were believed to have 'degeneration' as their main aetiological factor. Alzheimer did not deny that there were greater diagnostic difficulties in respect of the various types of 'endogenous' mental diseases, as compared to the 'organic' ones. However, in clear opposition to Hoche, he wanted to apply Kraepelin's concept of distinct entities to both groups, 'organic' as well as 'functional', while for the latter, he even postulated 'different stems of degeneration'.

Alzheimer summarised his pro-Kraepelinian point of view in the following, rather harsh critique of Hoche:

> 'What deeper medical knowledge about psychopathological states do we gain by establishing a paranoid, querulant, catatonic, melancholic symptom complex? Today, we already recognise such symptom complexes in very different diseases, and we know that some of them may occur in the same disease. . . . But it is my opinion that we would abandon our medical responsibility if we did not try to define their cause, course, or prognosis. We will, however, hardly be able to do so, if we do not succeed in detecting their relationship with a distinct disease process. So, by following Hoche's suggestion, we would cease the efforts to solve our most important problems, before having made the most of the means at our disposal.'[21]

In the same study, Alzheimer commented critically on the way scientific data were obtained in psychiatry. This represents a very 'modern' concept, decades before these issues again entered the mainstream of psychiatry, in the development of operationalised diagnostic criteria (e.g. DSM-III-R, ICD-10):

> 'What we urgently need in the field of mental disorder is an improvement in the way symptomatology is recorded. Today, casenotes are to some extent more a summary of judgements than of symptoms. Therefore, they are not scientific documents in a general sense, as some people still seem to believe, but in many respects subjective efforts, mirroring the personal opinions of the interviewer. This, of course, favours self-deception and makes it easy to provide us with presumed proofs for what was expected beforehand.'[21]

At the 1912 psychiatric meeting in Kiel, Hoche[81] once more criticised Kraepelin as 'the main proponent of classificatory optimism'. In his reply, Alzheimer repeated the arguments developed in his paper of 1910, adding that it was possible to bring forward further empirical evidence for Kraepelin's position. This was primarily through pathological anatomy, refining the assessment of clinical symptomatology and studies of aetiological factors; this should especially help to elucidate the relationship between symptom complexes and underlying disease processes. Sounding extraordinarily optimistic, Alzheimer claimed there was: 'justified hope that we will soon have established the anatomical basis of dementia praecox. . . . It is necessary, that we do not resign, but continue our work with all means.'[75]

In the discussion, Stransky spoke of 'Kraepelin's school', whose position did not seem incompatible with Hoche's. Kraepelin called the concept of distinct disease processes 'a useful heuristic idea', and Weygandt supported a critical assessment of psychiatric diagnoses, but at the same time warned of 'scepticism, which paralyses enthusiasm in research'[75].

Alzheimer was sceptical not only about Hoche's syndrome theory, but also about Carl Wernicke's localisation doctrine[82], which he believed to be too speculative, and not sufficiently corroborated by empirical data. He especially criticised the fact that it tended to over-estimate localising aspects, thus leading to an artificial classification. As a histopathologist, Alzheimer certainly admitted the relevance of exact topographical descriptions, but in a critical comment on Wernicke, he argued[65] that notwithstanding its importance for clinical symptomatology, it was not the localisation as such, but the localisation of a definite, i.e. distinct disease process in Kraepelin's sense, which constituted nosology. He repeatedly emphasised that Korsakow's psychosis and presbyophrenia[83], for example, may temporarily create the same clinical picture by affecting the same anatomical area. His subsequent argument was as much a Kraepelinian one, reminiscent of Karl Bonhoeffer's 1910 theory of the nosological non-specificity of psychopathological syndromes[84]. As Kraepelin probably would have put it, clinical similarities or differences are not useful tools for discovering the aetiology or nature of an underlying disease process. It is interesting how often both Kraepelin and Alzheimer used the term 'natural' with regard to psychiatric nosology, indicating their mutual aim to 'detect' the 'essence' (das Wesen) of distinct disease processes. Alzheimer's paper of 1912[66] and his following comment on Wernicke provide examples of this:

'Finally, we shall agree with Wernicke in assuming that the localisation of the disease process does have a nearly exclusive influence on the appearance of any given clinical picture of a mental illness. But let us consider the fact that the same disease process may manifest itself at different locations and that due to the identity of the disease process, these different foci show the same pathological development over time. In addition, we learn from the examples of presbyophrenia and Korsakow's psychosis that different disease processes may temporarily generate similar clinical pictures, because for some time they may have a similar localisation, whereas the difference between the disease processes themselves leads to a discrepancy in the further course of illness. Taking all this into account, it will be evident that we will develop a more natural classification of the various pathological states if we do not choose localisation, but the heterogeneity of histopathological processes as the basis for separating diseases from each other.'[65].

Alzheimer (and Nissl) had intended to produce empirical evidence in favour of Kraepelin's nosology, especially for his dichotomy between dementia praecox and manic-depressive illness, by means of histopathology. However, they did not succeed in this intention. Reports on histopathological findings in the cortex of psychotic patients remained heterogenous and contradictory, though at the same time, cerebral localisation continued to be a fast growing field of research; in 1918, the department of topographical histology was founded within the Munich Research Institute, K Brodmann being its first head.

For a long time, Alzheimer had been planning to write a comprehensive textbook about the histopathology of psychoses, thus summarising and critically reviewing the contemporary literature, as well as his own scientific work. But due to his early death in 1915—only three years after taking over the chair of psychiatry in Breslau— this plan could not be realised, apart from some preliminary concepts.

Alois Alzheimer's scientific work can be summarised briefly as follows: He favoured a 'medical' or, in a more modern term, 'biological' approach to psychiatric research. He emphasised that research should be firmly related to clinical questions. His personal and professional identity was that of a thoroughly educated and experienced clinician who was scientifically interested in histopathology. Conceptually, he took over Emil Kraepelin's basic positions concerning psychiatric nosology and the philosophical foundations of psychiatry.

Acknowledgement

I want to thank Alois Alzheimer's descendants, especially Mrs H Köppen, Wessling near Munich, for their valuable help, without which our knowledge about Alzheimer's life would be much smaller.

Chapter 4

Social Aspects of Alzheimer's Disease

H. L. Freeman

In the historical perspective, references to dementia can be found as early as the work of such classical authors as Solon, Plato, and Celsus[1], though the generally short expectation of life then must have made old age a relatively uncommon state. In the third and fourth Centuries AD, *gerontochia* for the care of the aged were established by the Eastern Church, and this responsibility was accepted to some extent later by the religious foundations of Western Europe[2]. After their Dissolution in England, however, poor houses were set up under the Law of 1601 which admitted some disabled old people, and the same was true in the American Colonies. The English Poor Law Amendment Act of 1834 was largely preoccupied with the able-bodied, but due to rapid population growth and industrialisation, the institutional system of workhouses that it established soon had to admit large numbers of the elderly. In 1909, though, the Minority Report of the Royal Commission on the Poor Law stated that out of the 140,000 old people contained by pauper Institutions, only 1000 were in any kind of special facilities, the rest being mixed with the sick, destitute, and handicapped of other age-groups. Ending life in the workhouse was a fate dreaded by the working classes, though one experienced all too often.

From the mid-nineteenth-century, voluntary and religious bodies also provided some accommodation for the aged in small homes, but even by 1944, this only amounted to about 9,000 places altogether in Britain. Townsend states that between 1910 and 1946, there was 'almost complete silence' on the subject in British publications and official enquiries, yet throughout this time the mental disability of old age was resulting in more and more admissions to mental hospitals. His own book, though, contains only one brief mention of senile dementia. Between 1931 and 1938, the number of people aged 65 and over admitted annually to mental hospitals in England and Wales rose from just under 3,000 to 3,850; in the latter year, the elderly accounted for 12% of all admissions and their admission rate, related to the aged population, was nearly double that for the population as a whole[3]. In 1900, 4.6% of the population of the United Kingdom was aged 65 years or more—a proportion which had reached 15% by 1985—whilst the general population grew from 38.2 to 56.5 million in that time. The mortality of those aged over

45 had only begun to decrease after about 1900, when birth rates also started falling in industrialised countries, though with a temporary rise in the 1950s and 60s.

In mid-nineteenth century Massachusetts and presumably in neighbouring states also, many of the insane remained confined in jails and almshouses, in spite of the growing populations within the state's three mental hospitals[4]. The elderly, though, seem to have suffered discrimination there based on age, since the total of them admitted to asylums did not grow proportionately with their numbers in the population. The explanation for this may be in the optimistic and curative image that asylums wished to project at that time, when most were fairly newly established, as well as in generally negative American attitudes towards the aged. Describing Worcester State Hospital in the early years of this century, Grob[5] states that any patient there who received a diagnosis of senile dementia on admission was immediately sent for permanent care to a custodial ward; the same fate befell those with diagnoses of dementia praecox or GPI.

In 1901, widely differing views on the care of senile dementia were expressed at a meeting of the Medico-Psychological Association of Great Britain and Ireland[6]. It was then a common complaint in asylum reports that they were becoming overcrowded by old people sent from workhouses and Poor Law infirmaries, so increasing asylum death rates and reducing the proportion of 'recoveries'. Dr DG Thomson estimated that the aged constituted 10-15% of asylum populations and that 'so far from being the placid, quiet old mental cyphers some would have us believe them to be', the majority showed 'all the symptoms of ordinary mental disorders *plus* special bodily and mental symptoms incidental to old age'. In his view, the county asylum was 'the proper receptacle for *all* cases of unsound mind occurring in the poor'; asylum care and treatment was necessary because of its 'elaborate structural arrangements and skilled nursing.' On the other hand, ordinary hospital or infirmary nurses neither could nor would manage such cases—'Nor can they be treated in the large open dormitories of hospitals or workhouses, where single-room accommodation and really good bathing arrangements, such as we know them in asylums, don't exist'. Though he admitted that 'asylums are far too elaborate and costly'— a view which it was no doubt politic for employees of local government to hold—Thomson said he knew of 'no part of an ordinary county asylum which could be done without in the treatment of senile cases except, perhaps, the buildings devoted to Divine worship, or to associated recreation'. On the other hand, 'in populous counties such as London, a special asylum, on cheaper lines than the ordinary asylum, might be set apart for senile cases'.

A much harder line came from Dr Robert Jones, who did not regard these patients as 'usually suffering from severe forms of insanity', and felt that 'the proper provision . . . is some sort of place where they can get the maximum amount of supervision for the minimum amount of cost'. Had there been old-age pensions (which were not in fact introduced until eight years later), 'some of these people might be cared for by their friends'. However, 'the great thing the workhouse authorities are afraid of is the frequent inquests that may take place after accidents have happened while these senile cases are under care, and therefore they wish to get rid of them to the asylum.' Dr D Bower agreed that 'senile manics' should only be treated in asylums, but that in the case of 'harmless senile dements', 'it would be a great hardship to remove them to the country asylum', rather than arranging for their care in their own homes or local workhouses. From Ireland, Dr MJ Nolan reported that an Act of three years earlier allowed the creation of 'auxiliary' asylums for chronic cases, which did not need to have medical or nursing staff and where the government grant would be only half that paid for asylum residents.

It is ironical that in the USA, UK, and similar countries, the 'whirligig of time' should have brought back this same solution for the care of the demented elderly in the 1970s and 1980s, with the process of deinstitutionalisation from mental hospitals to 'nursing homes'. Perhaps there are in fact very few basic strategies, when attempts are made to meet the problems of human societies, so that the same 'solution' will tend to be reinvented from one period to another. Burns et al.[7] found in samples from 112 US nursing homes that two-thirds of their residents were suffering from some psychiatric disorder, though funding systems discriminated against the elderly mentally ill and the expertise of both medical and other staff needed improving in this respect.

In a lecture of 1926, Dr GM Robertson[8] of the Royal Edinburgh Hospital emphasised the relationship between living conditions and the mental infirmities of old age: 'in the past there had been . . . a process of weeding out the less fit, before old age was reached, whereas at the present day there is an opposite process'. The result was an increase in both the numbers of the aged in proportion to the rest of the population and the total amount of insanity, since 'senility is the greatest insanity-producing period of life'. Robertson thought that syphilis and chronic alcoholism might be 'the essential agents in the causation of insanity late in life', whereas 'careful living in the middle period of life' was the best protective policy. In this respect, he was optimistic about the influence of sickness benefit, old-age pensions, improved housing, better sanitation, and a higher standard of living, but thereby was in fact somewhat self-contradictory, since all these would tend to prolong the expectation of life, and so cause what he had just identified as results which were undesirable epidemiologically.

In 1937, a highly innovative survey of all facilities which might be accommodating cases of psychiatric disorder in one city (Oxford) was undertaken by Dame Ellen Pinsent[9]. Even within this relatively small local authority, six different council committees had some responsibility for mental health, yet the whole situation was pervaded by a basic lack of interest in or understanding of psychiatric problems. The two hospitals for the indigent (Public Assistance Institutions) contained numbers of confused and incoherent old people, mixed up with the mentally retarded and psychotic, but no psychiatrist visited them, so that a proper diagnosis was never made. There seemed to be no real incentive to improve this situation amongst any of those concerned—whether professional or lay—and that situation remained largely unchanged for another decade.

During World War II, Sir Aubrey Lewis[3] reported a study of social factors in the admission of patients to a special mental hospital for the elderly—a subject which at that time attracted little scientific interest. The diagnoses for 50 consecutive admissions that Lewis studied were: senile dementia, 30; arteriosclerosis, 13; confusional state, 6; and pellegra, 1 (a surprising finding in London). Unravelling 'the tangle of medical and social threads that constitutes the later history of these wrecks', Lewis concluded that the majority had been ill-adjusted and difficult people for most of their lives. 'Loneliness, infirmities, disease, idleness, undernourishment, and poverty' had been common for them, but after hospital care, many could return to live in the community, 'provided always that the milieu will then be favourable to their social reintegration'. Lewis was forward-looking in emphasising the valuable contribution that could be made to the management of these cases by a skilled social worker—a contribution that is still unavailable in many services worldwide. Three years later, he drew attention to the vastly greater problems which an as yet unchanged psychiatric service would have to face from the inexorable rise in the numbers of old people during the second half of the century[10].

In 1948, responsibility for the demented elderly in Britain was rationalised, at least on paper, when those who were considered 'sick' were placed under the new National Health Service, and those 'in need of care and attention' under the new Welfare Departments of local authorities, which replaced Public Assistance arrangements (previously the Poor Law). The National Assistance Act of that year envisaged that workhouses would be replaced by small residential homes, while the Public Assistance Institutions for the sick poor had become NHS hospitals. This neat administrative solution did not always correspond with reality, though; sometimes a single building had to be divided up between two authorities, and with cases of dementia, arguments could go on endlessly as to whether these were the responsibility of welfare services, of psychiatry, or of medical geriatrics. Similar situations continue to be found in other industrialised countries.

However, led initially by a small band of enthusiasts, geriatric medicine began to develop as a specialty in Britain from 1948, and then became the most rapidly growing sector of medical care[11]. Some 20 years later, the sub-specialty of psycho-geriatrics started a similar trajectory, also acquiring a systematic training and academic cadre. A government circular of 1972[12] offered a rational basis for collaboration and for the distribution of functions between the different services involved, though it was less impressive in estimating the scale of resources needed for the mental illness of old age. From a service point of view, British geriatrics and psycho-geriatrics are at present the most advanced in the world, though similar developments are occurring in countries such as Australia and Switzerland[13], while the USA has a vast preponderance in basic research (*vide infra*).

In Newcastle-upon-Tyne, Kay *et al.*[14] found that the 6.2% of the elderly population which suffered from organic brain syndromes contributed 46% of the admissions to geriatric hospital beds; however, four out of five of the old people with these severe disorders were living at home. The total prevalence for elderly persons with psychiatric disorder within institutions was 17.1 per 1000, of whom nearly half had severe dementia and almost one-quarter mild dementia. However, in a more recent British survey, two-fifths of old people with moderate or severe dementia were living in residential homes or long-stay hospital wards[15]. The situation has been aptly described by Roth[16] as 'a precarious equilibrium between the large morbidity in the community and the small proportion of it that flows, ever so slowly, into institutional accommodation.' A detailed account of the development and organisation of the psycho-geriatric service for one-third of the city of Manchester has been given by Jolley & Jolley[13], though unfortunately, changes in both health and social services have since impaired its effectiveness. In Britain, hospital bed numbers have been consistently reduced over more than 30 years (with gathering momentum since the late 1980s), as the care of chronic disorders has been progressively removed from inpatient services. Cooper[17] points out that this transition from clinical to non-clinical residential care is 'more readily explained in socio-political terms than by any real improvement in the outcome (of dementia)'.

In Europe, WHO[18] has recommended that 'A medical/social service for old people should be organized on a district basis, and should include a psychogeriatric assessment unit'; long-term hospital care was seen as the last resort, but its prevention requires the integration of services at various levels, including primary medical care. Since those with dementia often need care rather than treatment, the primary requirement is for nursing, which should be available outside institutions (though it rarely is, in most countries); many sufferers could be managed well in caring facilities which do not have the full services of a hospital.

From their survey of the elderly in New York and London, Gurland *et al.*[19] concluded that increasing the volume of activity of any extramural service, e.g. domiciliary nursing, will not necessarily alter rates of admission to institutions. If, for instance, these services are commercially operated, they will clearly do everything they can to maintain their volume of activity. Therefore, a need exists to plan systems of care which provide a variety of options, operate in a flexible way, and project a reassuring and supportive image.

Yet even an ideal domiciliary service would be unable to support all people suffering from dementia at home indefinitely[20]. It has been widely hoped that early identification of cases, followed by the availability of packages of care designed to help impaired old people to remain at home, would greatly reduce the need for admission to institutions. Unfortunately, though, there is little firm evidence up to now that this can be achieved. In Cambridge, a multidisciplinary team was established for this purpose, with the participation of a geriatrician and psycho-geriatrician[21]. It offered a wide range of assistance, including extra finance, physical aids, domestic help, respite admissions, practical advice, family counselling, relatives' support groups, and night sitters. Amongst those subjects with moderate or severe dementia who lived with supporters, the intervention made no difference to the rate of admission to long-term care. However, amongst those who lived alone, significantly more of the intervention group than of the controls were admitted. The intervention seems to have had the paradoxical effect, therefore, of bringing forward the admission of demented subjects who lived alone because of earlier knowledge that they were seriously at risk. The authors suggest that with greater experience, the team might become more effective in helping people to continue living at home, but also with the passage of time, team members will inevitably change, so that some will always be relatively inexperienced in the work.

The emergence of Alzheimer's Disease

Fox[1] has analysed the scientific and social processes whereby 'from an obscure, rarely applied medical diagnosis, Alzheimer's Disease has emerged to become the fourth or fifth leading cause of death in the United States, in little more than 12 years'. Alliances between a few interested neuroscientists, the National Institute on Aging (NIA), an advocacy organisation, charitable foundations, and the media provided a focus for political action, which in turn generated enormous support for further research, but this required the construction of a unifying, disease-specific focus. Fox states that until the application of electron microscopy to neurological disorders in the early 1960s, Alzheimer's Disease had been considered a rare presenile condition; when evidence of neurochemical changes began to emerge, though, in the 1970s the condition became of wider scientific interest. The financial support for that interest derived from recognition by the National Institute on Aging of the importance of a disease-specific or 'categorical' approach; as a result, the research budget for this disorder increased by 800 times between 1979 and 1989. This would not have been possible, though, had the National Institutes of Health not provided 'a pre-existing social infrastructure that facilitated the aggregation of scientific, political and public resources for the development of a social movement.'

Fox also emphasises the importance of the proposal by Katzman and Karasu[22] that 'senile dementia' should be discarded as a diagnosis and these patients included in the category of Alzheimer's Disease. As a result, the number of potential cases in the population increased many times over and when estimates were made of the costs of long-term care for these, a strong argument developed for greater federal support for Alzheimer-related research. This connecting of 'senility' to a specific neurological disease meant a denial of the commonly held belief that growing old itself caused dementia, and the reconceptualisation which occurred then allowed collective action to be mobilised around what was now seen to be a significant social and health problem. From the scientific point of view, the availability of specific NIA grants, special conferences, opportunities for publication in new journals and books, and later the interest of large pharmaceutical companies all had the effect of directing research interest and research workers into what had previously been a generally neglected area. However, since complex scientific programmes do not produce results quickly, it was not to be until the later 1980s that significant new information began to emerge about Alzheimer's Disease, in such areas as genetics.

Epidemiological aspects
Epidemiology might provide a route to greater understanding of the aetiology and other still inscrutable aspects of Alzheimer's Disease. In fact, though, progress of this kind has been relatively slow, mainly because of the need for 'differential-diagnostic criteria, based on the phenomena of disease and validated again autopsy findings'[17]. The problem, as Cooper makes clear, is that 'primary degenerative dementia is essentially a diagnosis of exclusion, which cannot be definitely confirmed during life and, indeed, not always *post mortem*; that no biological marker is available for use in case identification and, finally, that neither for dementia of Alzheimer type nor for multi-infarct dementia is it yet clear whether we are dealing with a single disease entity or with the final common pathway of a number of different morbid processes.' Furthermore, counting the number of sufferers from dementia is problematic, since there is no universally agreed criterion for what constitutes 'a case' and there are particular difficulties at the less severe end of the spectrum[23].

Incidence and prevalence rates—whether for dementia as a whole or specifically for Alzheimer's Disease—are very difficult to measure, not least because many sufferers never come into contact with health or social services, even in countries where these are of a high standard: 'If the aim is to estimate the size of the problem for administrative purposes, then the definition should be linked to the need for particular services'[24]. Nevertheless, as Cooper[17] points out, the similarity between age-related curves from different studies does suggest that different investigators have been studying the same phenomenon. Mortimer et al.[25] calculated prevalence rates for specific types of dementia in the population aged 65 and over as: Alzheimer's Disease, 2.5%; multi-infarct dementia, 0.9%; combined forms, 0.9%; and other causes, 0.1%. These rates would not necessarily hold for general populations, though, because the relative sizes of the younger age-groups vary so widely between different countries and regions.

The relationship between pre-senile and senile dementia might be illuminated to some extent by better knowledge of incidence rates. Cooper[17] states that if these represented different nosological entities, then the corresponding age-specific incidence rates should follow a bimodal pattern, whereas if they are sub-groups of a single disease, separated only by an artificial cut-off of age, the distribution should be unimodal. The only data offering 'true' incidence rates for pre-senile dementia come from Israel[26], where there is a steep rise from 0.003 per 1000 at 40-44 years to 0.058 per 1000 at 55-59, representing a doubling in the rate for each extra 3-4 years of age. If this curve is extrapolated beyond the age of 60, it corresponds fairly well to rates of 'treated' incidence from several countries. Cooper regards this as providing some support for the view that Alzheimer's Disease is a single pathological process, which cannot satisfactorily be divided into sub-categories on the basis of age alone.

In their study comparing old people in New York and London, Gurland et al.[19] were surprised to find that prevalence rates of dementia were significantly higher in the former city, which could not be explained by diagnostic or demographic differences or by longer duration of illness; incidence rates were in the same direction. Between 2.5% and 5% of the community population aged 65 and over could definitely be diagnosed as suffering from dementia, while another 2.5% of the general elderly population were demented residents of institutions; in London, the overall proportion of the elderly population who were in institutions was slightly lower. Rates of dementia were about 20% in the population aged over 80.

In an attempt to compare the frequency of the two main forms of the disorder, Jorm et al.[24] analysed 47 published data sets, of which 18 presented some separation of rates into those for Alzheimer's Disease and multi-infarct dementia respectively: the actual levels of dementia reported varied greatly from one study to another. Their conclusion was that whilst true regional differences may exist, it is impossible to assess their extent from existing data, because of the many methodological differences between the studies. From those which give sufficient detail, though, it appears that rates for Alzheimer's Disease tend to be higher among females, whereas the opposite is true of multi-infarct dementia. In spite of the limitations of published studies, it does seem that there are significant regional differences, with Japanese and Russian investigations reporting higher rates for multi-infarct dementia, whereas all others (except one) showed either no significant difference or significantly higher rates of Alzheimer's Disease.

Two Asian studies throw some further light on these possible regional differences. Shibayama et al.[27] screened a random sample of 3106 community residents aged 65 and over in Aichi Prefecture, Japan for dementia. Prevalence rates for multi-infarct dementia and Alzheimer's Disease were given as 2.8% and 2.4% respectively (other forms were 0.6%); this did not seem to confirm the suggestion that multi-infarct is the predominant kind of dementia in that country, but it was diagnosed more often in men. Overall, a lower prevalence of dementia was found in city than in rural residents, though it was not known whether the age-structure of the population was different in the two kinds of area or whether impaired elderly people were more likely to be tolerated in less densely populated circumstances. From China, Shen et al.[28] reported a three-year follow-up study of 1090 people aged 60 or over in an urban area of Beijing. The prevalence rate of combined moderate and severe dementia was 1.1% in those aged 65 and over. In both incident and prevalent cases, the ratio of multi-infarct dementia to Alzheimer's Disease was 3:2, unlike the results of most studies from Europe and North America. Even within China, however, the ratios between the two appear to vary among different regions. In Shanghai, Zhang et al.[29] found a significantly higher prevalence rate of Alzheimer's Disease than of Multi-infarct Dementia among subjects aged 65 and over; this was consistent with a reported lower than average incidence rate of cerebral vascular disease in south China[30].

Indications of a possible secular trend towards changes in the rates of the two main forms of dementia have come from the Lundby epidemiological study in southern Sweden, over a 25-year period[31]. In the 1947-57 cohort, age-standardised prevalence rates for Alzheimer's Disease and multi-infarct dementia were 2.19 and 3.13% for men and 3.05 and 1.83% for women, in subjects aged 60 and over. For the 1957-72 sample, the rates were 2.13 and 5.3% for men and 2.35 and 2.32% for women. However, these trends for Alzheimer's Disease to become less common and multi-infarct dementia more common over time were not statistically significant and do not seem to have been confirmed elsewhere. Possibly the very high standard of living in Sweden might have resulted in some modest improvement of this kind.

The expected numbers of those with dementia in different regions and areas will clearly be related to general population trends and to factors such as migration. In Australia, where there was very large-scale immigration from the 1950s onwards, mainly of younger and middle-aged adults with children, the number of people with dementia is expected to double between 1981 and 2001 and to continue rising after this[31]. At present, half those with moderate or severe dementia there are in institutions—a situation rather different from that in the United Kingdom, for instance.

Risk factors

So far as risk factors are concerned, there are consistent findings that age is the most important one; prevalence rates of both multi-infarct dementia and Alzheimer's Disease double about every five years, the former rather more steeply. Jorm et al.[24] found only three studies giving enough data to allow consideration of differences in rates due to age, sex, and type of dementia: for Alzheimer's Disease, age-adjusted rates for females were significantly higher than those for males, whereas for multi-infarct dementia, there was no significant sex difference. A cohort of volunteer males was followed for 20 years by Sluss et al.[33], who found that the probability of escaping Alzheimer's Disease fell from 1.00 at the age of 60 to 0.71 at 85; thus, the very old, in whom the incidence of Alzheimer's is highest, are a survival population.

The influence of genetic factors in dementia is difficult to estimate without a better knowledge of its frequency among elderly people in the population. However, Larsson et al.[34] were among the earliest research writers to draw attention to the importance of family history, while Heston[35] found an extreme concentration of risk among the relatives of those in whom the disease started before the age of 65, particularly when one or both parents had also had the condition. Using the family history method, Mohs et al.[36] estimated the familial aggregation of Alzheimer's Disease in 50 first-degree relatives of probands, compared with 45 matched controls. Using a life-table method, the relatives showed a cumulative risk which was four times the control value, whereas the rates for spouses of probands were no different from those of the control groups. Environmental causes could not be entirely ruled out, but the data supported the operation of a relatively common dominant autosomal gene whose expression is delayed until late old age and largely completed by the age of 90. The estimation of familial risks can be very complex, but in general, they seem to be 'consistent with the hypothesis of Mendelian dominant genetic causes'[37].

In the search for possible environmental factors, suspicion has fallen on aluminium, neurotoxic amino-acids derived from various plants, viral infections, auto-immune reactions, and head injuries. Theoretically, various risk factors of this kind might share some final common path which would result in damage to the central nervous system, but no mechanism of this kind has yet been discovered. However, Roth[38] has proposed a clinical 'threshold' for dementia: the combination of damage from one or more environmental factors over the life-span might combine with age-related deterioration to bring forward the point at which there is functional decompensation and the person can be diagnosed as mentally impaired. In that case, the interval between exposure to the risk factor and the clinical onset of dementia might be expected to vary widely, which greatly increases the difficulty of investigating the question through epidemiological methods. This model would also provide an explanation for the fact that Alzheimer's Disease and multi-infarct dementia are not uncommonly found co-existing as a mixed disorder[39].

It has often been believed that social disadvantage in its various forms is a causative factor for psychiatric disorder, including dementia, though, there is 'no convincing evidence of a relationship between indices of underprivilege and the causation of mental disorder in old age'[15]. However, up to now, the subject has not been studied specifically to any great extent. Social factors are important, though, in influencing the likelihood of such people having to leave home to go into institutional care, as Lewis had pointed out in his wartime study (vide supra). Such general social changes as greater mobility of the population, the break-up of extended families, and the increased tendency for women to work outside the home are all likely to make community care of mentally impaired old people more difficult.

From the sociological viewpoint, Busfield[40] condemns the present methods of dealing with the problem of dementia, which offer care and treatment to specific individuals who have been medically identified as demented, while research underpins this type of intervention by concentrating on physical changes in the brain. On the other hand, little attempt is said to have been made to look at factors such as 'social isolation, the lack of family and social support, and the lack of material resources, meaningful work and status (which) may . . . make it difficult for the growing numbers of those aged over 65 to lead independent lives; and may help to generate dependence, distress and confusion which may . . . make a diagnosis of dementia more likely'. Busfield goes on to suggest that social intervention which aimed to strengthen and ensure the independence of the over-65s 'would arguably do more for that group as a whole than simply trying to cope with the ever increasing numbers of those already identified as demented'.

This argument assumes that Alzheimer's Disease could be confronted with the same preventive model as infectious diseases such as cholera—that (figuratively) our resources are being used to treat infected cases symptomatically, rather than cut off the source of polluted water. But dementia has not yet found its John Snow. The short passage quoted above contains the word 'may' three times, as well as an 'arguably'; it does not rest on a single demonstrated fact. It is perfectly true that even the wealthiest society could not care for all cases of dementia through medical and social services. It is equally true that fostering the independence of elderly people is a socially valuable goal which deserves its share of public expenditure. The assumption, though, that pursuing the second policy would make the first unnecessary rests on no foundation whatever.

Exactly the same reasoning was used by Caplan[41] in his approach to psychiatric disorder in general. He advocated concentrating resources on interventions by people who were not mental health professionals with members of the population affected by personal crises. Specialist personnel were to have a mainly educative and consultative role. Again, the assumption was that such 'preventive' efforts would greatly reduce the amount of serious psychiatric disorder in the population at risk. Again, no evidence was provided that this was likely to happen and again, no advice was offered as to how those already affected by illness or disability were to be dealt with, once resources had been removed from their treatment and care. Although enormously influential in the 1960s and 70s, these views now have few adherents[42]. No one would deny that the social context of dementia is very important from every point of view, but if a truly 'preventive' form of intervention is to be found, this seems most likely to be through the activities of biological scientists.

Chapter 5

The Vascular Dementias

T. R. Dening and G. E. Berrios

Current accounts of vascular dementia[1] tend to identify the paper by Hachinski *et al.*[2] as the moment in which the old notion of 'arteriosclerotic dementia' was replaced by the new paradigm of 'multi-infarct'. However, since the history of these disorders has attracted relatively little attention, this may be questionable, and the novelty of the multi-infarct paradigm more apparent than real.

The view that a state of dementia might result from changes in the blood supply to the brain, rather than from primary changes in its tissues, developed fully only during the 1870s. For this, five important conceptual components were needed: 1, a stable clinical description of dementia; 2, a pathophysiology of the cerebral blood supply; 3, a relationship between brain function and structure; 4, a model of nervous tissue to differentiate between the effects of primary and secondary cell distress; and 5, a model of changes due to ageing. Each of these components has a different history and chronology; other chapters in this book deal with the clinical notion of dementia but the history of the other four will be explored here.

Cerebral circulation

Anatomical knowledge of cerebral supply was obtained earlier than understanding of its physiology. During the middle of the seventeenth century, after the work of Jakob Wepfer and particularly of Thomas Willis, the basic anatomical idea was clarified of four main arteries joined together by a basal arterial circle[3]. Details on the dynamic aspects of this closed system, however, took longer to emerge. For example, there was much eighteenth-century debate as to whether, given that the skull was a rigid box, there could be a variation in the total volume of blood circulating through the brain. That there could not was suggested by Alexander Monro (The Second), the great Scottish anatomist[4,5], and provided with some empirical evidence by his disciple George Kellie. The Monro-Kellie 'doctrine' held sway until the mid-nineteenth century, when the Dutch scientist Cornelis Donders developed his 'window' technique to show that changes in blood volume did, in fact, take place and that these might be related to variations in blood pressure and in the rate of respiration. It was also suggested that the observed vasoconstriction was mediated by localised autonomic nervous system control, but this view was challenged by Leonard Hill[6] and for more than 20 years, the subject was diverted into a cul-de-sac.

Further debate concerned the extent to which the arterial anastomosis was dynamically sufficient to deal with sudden drops in blood supply which affected any of the four participating vessels, as well as the even more complex issue of whether or not cortical arterioles were terminal, in which case there would be regions which were vulnerable to major reductions in blood supply. Views on cerebral physiology, in turn, influenced the development of theories of brain softening during the nineteenth century.

Relationship between brain function and structure

As other chapters in this book have made clear, organic theories of dementia, in the modern sense of 'organic', only developed during the nineteenth century. The assumption that certain mental and physical states might be related to general disturbances in the nervous system—the neuralpathology doctrine—had appeared during the previous century[7]. All the *neuroses* were 'organic' disorders, in that the 'sense and movement' (vibration) of the nervous system was believed by Cullen to be compromised in many diseases[10], but the nineteenth century moved away from this kind of abstract thinking. 'Organic' came to mean focalised structural damage, so that for the first time, some dementias were identified as truly organic. Examples included the chronic arachnoiditis state described by Bayle[8], and the various disorders of psychological collapse described by Léon Rostan in association with softening of the brain[9] (*vide infra*).

However, as the century progressed, the states of dementia associated with the insanities (vesanic dementias) became a difficult classificatory problem. Due to persistent failures to find neuropathological changes, the realisation became stronger that many of the insanities might not be accompanied by abnormalities in the brain. The vesanic dementias also created a serious problem in that although post-mortem studies of elderly patients showed changes (no different from those seen in the normal elderly), young subjects with vesanic dementia did not. Together with the gradual narrowing of the concept of dementia itself, this difficulty led to the eventual discarding of the vesanic dementias from the group of the true dementias, and the creation, at the end of the century, of the concept of pseudodementia.

Models of nervous tissue

Understanding of the clinical states of brain softening, stroke, and eventually arteriosclerotic dementia depended on the development of models whereby tissue distress, due to reduction in blood supply, might be expressed. Whether the mental changes in vascular dementia directly resulted from cell death (related to acute episodes of stroke) or from chronic reductions in blood supply (independent of strokes) was the crucial issue. Since the early nineteenth century, each view had received fluctuating support. Both Rostan[11] and Durand-Fardel[12] held that long-term cognitive deficit in subjects with 'white softening' results from strokes. Durand-Fardel stated that: 'when softening occurs as the result of a stroke, or a series of strokes, cognition (*intelligence*) is more markedly affected and the patient falls into dementia (*hébétude absolue*)' (p328). However, as the notion of atheroma and arteriosclerosis developed, a second view emerged—that restriction in the lumen of vessels might lead to a chronic reduction of blood supply and thus cause a corresponding reduction in mental functioning. This view gained momentum as the century progressed[13].

Brain changes with ageing

In the present century, there have been two schools of thought on arteriosclerotic dementia. The first was that the dementia resulted from cell death, age only being relevant as a factor in the development of strokes; the second view was that age was the central factor in the development of arteriosclerosis and hence of the dementia that followed. Therefore, the debate depended to some extent on theories of arteriosclerosis[14], which became a favourite explanation amongst the supporters of the notion of 'senile insanity'. According to this, ageing imposed particular clinical characteristics upon certain psychiatric diagnoses, e.g. predicted a bad outcome in involutional melancholia. Although even Kraepelin sympathised with this view for a while, it was challenged by Walton[15], who stated that arteriosclerosis was not an important factor in the aetiology and prognosis of the involutional psychoses. The idea, however, retained some support until the time of the Second World War, when Mayer-Gross again called it into question[16].

Dementia and brain softening

Cases of brain 'softening' accompanied by cognitive failure were described since the early nineteenth century; Rostan, for example, described 98 cases which he thought were scorbutic in origin[17]. He suggested three types of softening—simple, abnormal, and complicated; psychiatric changes could follow either abnormal or complicated softening, and might occur before, during, or after the softening itself. Thus, senile dementia and insanity might precede softening, but Rostan wondered whether they were simply 'latent' manifestations of the disorder. He described major changes associated with stroke, such as a marked drop in intelligence and acute insanity, but claimed that these could not be used to locate the area of softening: 'they are a general sign . . . not a positive sign of localisation' (pp214-215).

Concerning the relationship between softening and insanity, Durand-Fardel[18] pointed out that 'softening' was being used to refer both to a *disease* (stroke) and to a *state* of the brain. He divided the psychiatric complications of cerebral accidents into acute and long-term—acute complications included confusion, depression, irritability, acute insanity, and loss of all the mental faculties (p139), while chronic complications were characterised by gradual onset, impaired memory, poverty of thinking, and a regression to infantile forms of behaviour; either could lead to 'true dementia' (pp327–328). Hughlings Jackson stated that the use of 'softening . . . as a category for a rude clinical grouping was to be deprecated' (p335)[19]. He followed Durand-Fardel's classification and described three types of mental symptoms: direct, following after few hours, and occurring after months. Jackson recognised the major cognitive failure that might ensue, and interpreted it in terms of his model of 'dissolution'[20]. Emotional symptoms were considered as release phenomena, while anxiety, stress, and irritability were listed as the most common clinical features that might precede stroke.

Apoplectic dementia

However, it was in the work of Benjamin Ball (1881), a French professor of British origin, that the notion of 'apoplectic dementia' became fully formed. Bell defined 'organic apoplexy' as a condition which may result from bleeding, softening, or tumour, any of which 'might be followed by a notable drop in cognition, and by a state of dementia which was progressive and incurable . . . of the three, localised softening (*ramollissement en foyer*) causes the more severe states of cognitive impairment' (p581)[21]. Ball believed that months before the actual stroke, the patient may experience prodromal features such as temporary lapses of cognition and sensory symptoms, caused by the atheromatous lesions affecting brain circulation. Particularly telling are episodes of somnolence and confusion, during which there is automatic behaviour and of which no memory exists after the event, as well as visual hallucinations, occasionally of a pleasant nature. After the stroke, persistent cognitive impairment is the commonest psychiatric symptom. Postmortem studies in these cases often showed softening of specific 'ideational' areas of the cortex, but also lesions in white matter.

Ball also believed that there was a laterality effect (p582), in that strokes affecting the right hemisphere gave rise more often to dementias with intellectual impairment, whereas those affecting the left hemisphere tended to cause perplexity, apathy, and unresponsiveness, and these subjects often talked to themselves. Such 'tranquil dementias' were often accompanied by aphasia. Left hemisphere lesions might also cause a 'special excitation of the emotional faculties, maudliness, involuntary laughter, and suicidal behaviour' (p583), and Ball followed Luys in the view that these symptoms resulted from specific damage to the corpus striatum, the insular sulci, and the temporal lobe. He also expressed surprise at their 'paradoxical' nature—that local cortical destruction may sometimes lead to loss of a function and sometimes to an exaggeration of it. He agreed with Luys that this might be due to modulation of emotional excitation by the temporal lobe.

Also during Ball's time, increasing emphasis was placed on red rather than white softening. Charcot (1881) wrote forcibly in favour of 'cerebral haemorrhage' (a term he proposed for red softening), which he suggested was commonly caused by diffuse arteriosclerosis: 'having eliminated all these cases, we find ourselves in presence of a homogeneous group corresponding to the most common form of cerebral haemorrhage. This is, par excellence, sanguineous apoplexy . . . as it attacks a great number of old people, I might call it senile haemorrhage, if it was not for the fact that it may be found with the same characters at the other periods of life' (p267)[22].

The formation of the concept of arteriosclerotic dementia

By the early twentieth century, psychiatrists had incorporated the diagnosis of arteriosclerotic dementia into the wider category of 'mental disorders of cerebral arteriosclerosis' (e.g. Barret, 1913[23]). Arteriosclerosis could be general or localised to the nervous system, and was caused by factors such as inheritance, atheroma, syphilis, alcohol, nicotine, high blood pressure, and age. The cerebral arteries were considered to have less elasticity than others in the body and to be thinner in genetically predisposed individuals. Arteriosclerosis caused mental changes both directly through narrowing of arteries, and indirectly through reactive inflammation in the nervous tissue, leading to four characteristic types of pathology: focal brain atrophy, subcortical encephalitis (i.e. Binswanger's disease—dealt with elsewhere in this book), perivascular gliosis, and senile cortical devastation (pp682-683).

By this period, the characteristic view that arteriosclerotic dementia was due to a gradual strangulation of blood supply to the brain had formed. Hence, much more emphasis was given to the prodromal symptoms than in the time of Rostan and Durand-Fardel, 100 years before. The actual stroke, when it finally came, was seen as the culmination of a process started many years before.

Marie (1906) offered an explanation for the popularity of arteriosclerosis as a mechanism—that it had been adopted by many as a general explanation of ageing[24]. Thus, Lancereux had developed the idea of a generalised arteritis, and Gull suggested that a number of cardiac and renal diseases resulted from arteriosclerosis. Marie accepted these views with some reservation, though, suggesting that 'there was in this explanation a sort of vicious circle: ageing is caused by arteriosclerosis, the latter by ageing' (p358). Likewise, pathologists studying 'senile dementia' worried because they could not 'safely exclude cerebral arteriosclerosis of greater or less degree in any single case' (p677)[25]. The great neuropsychiatrist Gustav Olah (1910) asked what specifically was meant by the term 'arteriosclerotic psychoses', arguing that there was no such category in the sense of having a clinical individuality and specific anatomical findings. All that there seemed to be was a progressive form of dementia, usually fatal, apparently connected with cerebral arteriosclerosis and generally related to motor symptoms[26].

The same approach was taken in the Textbook (1915) edited by Binswanger, Hoche et al, where a section was dedicated to mental disorders caused by arteriosclerosis[27]. The German writers also felt that the genetic component was important, and identified three types of arteriosclerotic condition: neurotic (including disorders of mood and neurasthenia), epileptic, and the dementias, which they characterised both as disturbance of cognition and of mood, occasionally leading to suicidal ideas. This account concentrated on two of the three types of arteriosclerotic change—chronic subcortical encephalitis, and perivascular gliosis. Both disorders were said to have a bad prognosis.

However, the view that arteriosclerotic dementia was not necessarily mediated by strokes continued in the 'chronic global ischaemia' hypothesis. For example, North and Bostock (1925), in a series of 568 cases from two mental hospitals, found that around 40% were suffering from arterial disease. They believed that this might account for the various mental conditions described; for example, in young schizophrenics, the link might be provided by an 'effete germ-plasm—an abiotrophy' leading also to arterial pathology[28]. Claude (1922) described white, red, and yellow softening and suggested that this condition led more often to dementia: 'the course of softening is unfavourable. In the young subject the rule is the one episode, in the elderly successive episodes . . . which lead to a specific picture which include a short-steps gait, memory failure, apathy, urinary incontinence, hemiplegia, and cognitive collapse' (p109)[29]. In 1927, Claude went further and suggested that in some cases, there could be 'cerebral starvation' with focal signs[30].

The aftermath
By the 1940s, the notion of arteriosclerotic dementia was fully formed, and was accepted in most countries. Vallejo Nagera (1945), for example, in a popular textbook described it in specific terms: compared with senile dementia it was more common in males, with more neurological signs. Two arteriosclerotic lesions were recognised: atheromatosis (affecting large vessels) and arteriosclerosis (affecting small vessels). Following Alzheimer and Spielmeyer, he divided the parenchymal lesions caused by these mechanisms into three groups: large focal softenings (seen at any age), multiple lacunar degenerations

(typical of the elderly), and irregular miliary foci (also common in the elderly). The prodromal period of the arteriosclerotic insanity might last for years and was characterised by fatigue, irritability, headaches, occasionally disinhibited behaviour, and personality disorders that might lead to conflict with the law. Focal motor and sensory signs were not the rule and were almost always transient. The second stage of the disease included the development of a state of dementia with some specific features, such as maudliness, emotional incontinence, delusions and hallucinations, panic attacks, and confabulations, all the florid symptomatology becoming fragmented and then disappearing as the dementing stage progressed. Terminal emaciation and infections led to death, but episodes of stroke, with concomitant motor sequelae, were rare[31].

This description is typical of the way the condition of arteriosclerotic dementia appeared up to the 1960s, and is markedly different from the definition of 'vascular or multi-infarct' dementia which was to develop in the middle 1970s, and be incorporated in ICD-9: 'dementia attributable, because of physical signs [on examination of the central nervous system] to degenerative arterial disease of the brain. Symptoms suggesting a focal lesion of the brain are common. There may be a fluctuating or patchy intellectual defect with insight, and an intermittent course is common. Clinical differentiation from senile or presenile dementia, which may coexist with it, may be very difficult or impossible' (p23)[32]. It is possible that this recent conceptual shift reflects the history of brain imaging technology, and in particular the introduction of computerised tomography[33]—a technique which excels at demonstrating anatomical lesions. Conceivably, further advances in techniques of measurement of cerebral blood flow may stimulate a revival in the fortunes of the 'global ischaemia' hypothesis.

Thus in current terminology, the contribution of focal lesions resulting from strokes has been emphasised, rather than that of potentially reversible generalised ischaemia. That this debate is not new has been shown above. An important question for the historian is whether arteriosclerotic dementia has disappeared from current classifications because present clinicians deny that the symptom-complex that once characterised it ever existed, or because they reject the notion of chronic global cerebral ischaemia that was believed to cause it. The literature is not clear about this. For example, Marshall (1988), in answering the question: 'Vascular and multiple dementia, do they exist?' states that 'multiple infarcts are not the only cause of vascular dementia. Low cerebral blood flow with diffuse cerebral ischaemia can develop as a result of severe extracranial occlusive disease . . . occasionally . . . patients present with a form of dementia resulting from low perfusion . . . ' (p3)[34]. Tomlinson & Corsellis (1984), on the other hand, categorically state: 'No good evidence exists, however, for a dementing syndrome resulting from chronic global cerebral ischaemia, whether on clinical grounds or on neuropathological studies.' (p987)[35].

Whether rejecting the condition or its putative mechanisms, it appears that investigators have played down the specific nature of the symptomatology so clearly described in the past. It is currently asserted that multi-infarct (vascular) dementia is uncommon, comprising between 10 and 15% of cases, or that the symptoms described result from a combination of multiple infarcts and Alzheimer's disease. Several questions remain to be answered: Was the clinical description of arteriosclerotic dementia achieved simply because focal symptoms were ignored? Is there a similarity between the old symptom-cluster in question and the recently discovered 'frontal dementias'[36], 'subcortical dementias'[37] and 'progressive supranuclear palsies'[38]? Are these latter clinical categories simply new names for the old forms of arteriosclerotic dementia? Many of the answers to such questions will be empirical, but in some cases will be conceptual, i.e. to be explained as a change in the paradigm controlling clinicians' perceptions of a symptom-cluster that refuses to disappear.

Chapter 6

The History of Subcortical Dementia

C. Cahn

'Dementia' is a word that has undergone a number of semantic changes over the past several centuries as described by Berrios[1-3] in this volume. It had a much broader meaning in earlier periods, but throughout the centuries implied the existence of intellectual and behavioural deterioration associated with organic brain disease. 'Subcortical' clearly refers to the anatomical structures of the brain located under the cortex, but since the cerebral cortex is closely connected with subcortical structures, lesions in the one are very likely to affect the function of the other. As it is not yet possible to be very precise in describing what is and what is not 'subcortical dementia', the account given here should be considered tentative, incomplete, and possibly even controversial.

The history of the term
Although the term 'subcortical dementia' came into general use only in the 1970s, it appeared for the first time in 1932: a paper by von Stockert was entitled *Subcorticale Demenz*[4]. Oddly enough, though, it appears nowhere else in the paper, which concerned a post-encephalitic thought disturbance in a patient who showed none of the motor signs of parkinsonism[5]. In describing memory disorder, slowness, personality change, and disturbance of affect, von Stockert attributed the syndrome to a lesion in the substantia nigra. Though many other papers appeared in subsequent years describing various dementia syndromes related to subcortical lesions, these were without 'subcortical' and 'dementia' being juxtaposed.

However, it was as late as 1973 that 'subcortical dementia' was reintroduced by McHugh in an unpublished paper where he described the mental impairment occurring in Huntington's chorea with the term[6]. A year later, Albert *et al* used it to describe the intellectual deterioration of progressive supranuclear palsy. From then on, 'subcortical dementia' appears more and more frequently in the scientific literature, but is still not to be found in the glossaries of ICD-9[7] nor of DSM III-R[8].

Cardinal features
The cardinal features of subcortical dementia have been described by Cummings and Benson[9] as; forgetfulness, slowing of mental processes, intellectual deterioration characterised by impaired ability

to manipulate acquired knowledge, and personality and affective changes including apathy and depression. Elementary linguistic, calculating, and learning processes are intact, but use of stored information, ability to generate problem-solving strategies, and insight are impaired. In contrast to cortical dementia, aphasia, amnesia, and agnosia are absent, and the intellectual impairment is less pronounced.

A list of the diseases in which subcortical dementia is present can start with those in which it is primarily the subcortical grey matter that is affected (e.g. degeneration of the caudate nucleus in Huntington's disease, depigmentation of the substantia nigra in Parkinson's disease). Then, those diseases in which the principal lesions are in the white matter (e.g. periventricular atrophy in Binswanger's disease) can be added, but in many conditions, there is a mixture of lesions in both kinds of subcortical matter, and in some (certain vascular dementias), those and the cortex.

In fact, the cerebral cortex, the subcortical grey matter, and the association tracts between them function as a whole, so that a lesion in one usually affects the activities of the others. This has led some authors to question the validity of the concept of 'subcortical dementia', and the issue has not been settled even today.

Mayeux *et al*[6] reported a quantitative neuropsychological assessment of patients with Alzheimer's, Parkinson's, or Huntington's diseases, finding that the patterns of brain impairment were not distinct enough in the three disorders to warrant the existence of subcortical dementia as an entity separate from cortical dementia. They concluded that the neuropathological basis of dementia in all these diseases may result from a combination of cortical and subcortical degeneration. Whitehouse[10] quoted several studies in which a mixed picture emerged; for instance, in Alzheimer's disease, usually regarded as a typically cortical dementia, there are important lesions in the nucleus basalis of Meynert, in the locus ceruleus, in the raphe nucleus, and in the amygdala, while many patients with Parkinson's or Huntington's disease had significant cortical changes, indistinguishable from those seen in Alzheimer's disease. However, more recently, authors such as Cummings and Benson[9] have made a case for subcortical dementia as an 'emerging concept', which helps to differentiate the types of dementia that occur with different lesions in the brain. More research is needed, however, to clarify the role that both cortical and subcortical structures play in the production of the clinical signs and symptoms of dementia.

Assuming that the concept of subcortical dementia is useful enough to be retained, those disorders in which the pathological process is located primarily in the subcortical areas and in which dementia is a prominent feature will now be considered.

Diseases manifesting symptoms of subcortical dementia

Cummings and Benson[9,11] divide the subcortical dementias into those conditions, mostly degenerative in nature, which result in prominent movement disorder as well as intellectual deterioration, and others, mostly of vascular, infectious, toxic, or neoplastic origin, which are less selective in the way they affect the brain, producing mixtures of cortical and subcortical features.

The first group includes: Parkinson's disease, Huntington's disease, Wilson's disease, Hallervorden-Spatz disease, idiopathic calcification of the basal ganglia, thalamic dementia, Parkinson-dementia complex of Guam, spinocerebellar degenerations, progressive supranuclear palsy, and progressive subcortical gliosis. Examples of the second group are Binswanger's disease and the lacunar state (which are subcortical varieties of multi-infarct dementia); postencephalitic parkinsonism, carbon monoxide poisoning, and certain primary and metastatic neoplasms. The list is by no means complete. As the lesions in these conditions are rarely confined to subcortical structures, there may be a great variety of symptoms in addition to the dementia of subcortical type.

Antecedent history

Our present concept of subcortical dementia being a relatively recent one, it is not surprising that it has a long antecedent history: concepts of brain stem dementia and subcortical stimulation can be traced back to the Renaissance[5]. Throughout the nineteenth century, though, most studies on disorders which are now recognised as having primary involvement of subcortical structures had placed the emphasis on cortical damage as the major pathological process. Prominent neuropsychiatrists of that century such as Griesinger (1817-1868) and Meynert (1833-1892) did not succeed in identifying these relationships correctly. Griesinger tried to classify divergent clinical aspects of dementia, but his concept of the disorder was much broader than ours, while Meynert developed a model of brain function in which psychiatric symptoms were related to imbalances in blood flow in the cortical and subcortical structures[10]. Meynert extended his theories beyond what his anatomical studies and clinical observations could support, and was strongly criticised by his contemporaries Kraepelin and Nissl for creating a 'speculative brain mythology'.

In the early part of this century, Eugen Bleuler[12] described a symptom constellation including slowness of thinking, memory disorder, and behavioural disturbances, associated with demonstrable (or presumed) brain pathology, which he called *Psychoorganisches Syndrom*. However, neither he nor his son, Manfred Bleuler[13], who described the 'chronic amnestic syndrome', differentiated clearly between cortical and subcortical pathology.

In 1922, during the encephalitis pandemic, Naville[14] described a syndrome that was 'completely new, found in no other organic, psychiatric or functional illness, except perhaps in a few cases of classical parkinsonism'. Its main features were reduction in voluntary attention, spontaneous interest, initiative, and capacity for work and effort, along with fatiguability and some mild loss of memory. Naville named this *la bradyphrenie*—a form of psychomotor retardation which was a sequela of encephalitis, even when not preceded by the classical somnolent lethargy. Referring to Naville's role in the history of subcortical dementia, Mandell and Albert[5] state that he had described more or less the same syndrome as McHugh and Albert *et al* did over 50 years later.

Below, an attempt will be made to present in chronological order historical descriptions of various sometimes quite unusual conditions, which have been reported as underlying subcortical dementia; these conditions are not necessarily related to one another.

Parkinson's Disease
In 1817, James Parkinson wrote his now famous *Essay on the Shaking Palsy*[15,16], based on six cases, only three of which he had examined in detail. This was written when he was aged 62, and was the nineteenth of his 23 scientific publications. 'Parkinson's essay sharply illuminated a clinical entity which had been only dimly apprehended before. . . . The symptoms had previously been confused with a number of nosologically quite different maladies, including chorea, torsion spasms, forms of cerebellar disease, senile and alcoholic tremor, and even multiple sclerosis. The fact that his essay broke new ground is amply proved by the reviews in contemporary medical journals, which made it plain from the length of the quotations that what he had to say was quite new and unfamiliar . . . The essay is a superb model of lucid clinical description'[17].

Parkinson thought that the pathological site was in the spinal cord, with extension to the medulla oblongata as the disease progressed. It was not until 60 years later that Charcot applied the term *la maladie de Parkinson*, by which it has been known ever since. As for the dementia associated with the extrapyramidal symptoms of the disease, Parkinson at first stated that 'the senses and intellect [are] uninjured', but his case histories detailed the presence of mental disturbances. It is now generally accepted that about one-third to one-half of patients with Parkinson's disease show mild-to-moderate dementia of the subcortical kind, with slowness of response, deterioration of abstraction and concept formation, failure to initiate activities spontaneously, and impaired or slowed memory, but without aphasia, agnosia, or severe amnesia unless there is coexisting cortical pathology.

James Parkinson (1755-1824)

Born in the London suburb of Shoreditch, Parkinson lived and practised medicine there all his life; he took over his father's practice, as did one of his sons who succeeded him some years later. Parkinson became concerned with the problems of the poor, their inadequate health care, the lack of education for their children, and the miseries brought to all classes by war. He became a social reformer and political activist, publishing a dozen or so pamphlets on the injustices of his time, which were widely distributed. He also became an expert geologist and palaeontologist. In the medical field, Parkinson wrote widely on many different subjects such as appendicitis, gout, hydrophobia, dangers of sports, preservation of health and, of special interest to psychiatrists, 'Observations on the Act Regulating Madhouses'[18,19]. This was prompted by a painful experience of his own in which he was accused of having wrongfully certified a woman as insane; he drew attention to the need to reform the legislation, pointing out the difficulties of defining insanity and distinguishing cerebral diseases and personal eccentricities that could simulate mental illness. This monograph contributed to the Act of 1811, partly reforming the incarceration of the insane, which at least opened the door to improvements in what had often been a sorry situation.

Huntington's Disease

In 1872, George Huntington wrote a paper 'On Chorea'[20]. He stated later that he had simply given a description of that peculiar form of chorea that was quite prevalent at the east end of Long Island, New York. However, at least five others had preceded Huntington in describing the disease named after him. According to Hayden[21], the first definite mention of heredity in the causation of adult chorea was made in 1832 by the physician Elliotson. In a lecture on St Vitus's dance, published in *The Lancet*, he noted that when 'it occurs in adults it is frequently connected with paralysis or idiotism and will perhaps never be cured. . . . I have often seen it hereditary'[22]. In 1841, shortly after his graduation from Jefferson Medical College, Charles O Walters consulted his professor of medicine, Robley Dunglison, concerning 'the nature of a singular convulsive affection which prevailed in a part of the country with which he was familiar'. Dunglison (1842) printed Walters' letter in full in the first edition of his book on the practice of medicine; this description is almost as lucid as that of Huntington, 31 years later[23]. Another account was given in 1846 by Charles Gorman of Philadelphia as part of his doctoral dissertation before the Faculty of Jefferson Medical College. The original thesis was lost, but in 1848, Dunglison included this account in the third edition of his textbook[24]. In 1860, the Norwegian physician Johan Christian Lund gave a very accurate description of the disease; the account was in Norwegian, and was translated into English by Orbeck* only in 1959. In Norway, the disease is still sometimes referred to as 'Lund-Huntington's chorea'. A further description in 1863 was by Irving W Lyon, when he was a house physician at Bellevue Hospital in New York City. He too recognised the hereditary nature of the condition, writing that the people among whom it occurred had been known to interdict marriages between their children. Locally, the disease was considered to be a disgrace, perhaps because its origin was ascribed 'to a visitation upon those who had reviled and mimicked our Saviour while undergoing crucifixion, [thus] they and their children were ever after affected with choreal irregularities'[25]. Lyon described three cases, without being aware of the previous observations of Walters, Gorman, and Lund. Nor did Huntington give any references in his paper, except to a George B Wood who, as professor of medicine at the University of Pennsylvania, had mentioned three similar cases in his treatise on the practice of medicine published in 1855[26].

In spite of his lack of priority, Huntington's account of the disease was the most complete that had been made[27]; he clearly described the mental symptoms of the disease and the risk of suicide, as well as its progressive downhill course. By 1887, Huntington's work was well known in Germany, where Huber first referred to the disease as *Huntington'sche Chorea*[28].

George Huntington (1850-1916)
Born in East Hampton, Long Island, Huntington followed in his grandfather's and his father's footsteps in practising medicine; as a youngster, he had accompanied his father on his professional rounds and had seen his first case of 'that disorder'. Following graduation from the College of Physicians & Surgeons in 1871, he joined his father in practice and continued to observe the cases of the hereditary chorea. After moving to Ohio later that year, he read his first paper on chorea before the Meigs & Mason Academy of Medicine at Middleport. In 1874, he settled in New York and, except for two years in North Carolina, spent the remainder of his life in the practice of medicine in Dutchess County. Speaking before the New York Neurological Society in 1909, Huntington reminisced about his vivid memory of driving with his father through a wooded road, when they suddenly came upon two women, mother and daughter, both tall, thin, almost cadaverous, both bowing, twisting and grimacing. From this point on his interest in the disease never wholly ceased, although he had seen no further cases during the 37 years since he had written his original paper. He died in 1916 at the age of 66[21].

The fact that Bruyn *et al*[29] were able to identify over 2,000 references to Huntington's chorea in the scientific literature during

---

*Mentioned by Hayden (1987) without further reference

the 100 years' period from 1872 to 1972 attests to the tremendous interest that this disease has evoked all over the world.

Binswanger's Disease

In 1894 Otto Binswanger, professor of psychiatry at the University of Jena, published a paper on the differential diagnosis of general progressive paralysis; he briefly described eight patients with dementia who at autopsy were found to have pronounced atrophy of the white matter as well as severe cerebral arteriosclerosis. Although the condition came to be known as 'subcortical arterio-sclerotic encephalopathy', Binswanger himself named it *encephalitis subcorticalis chronica progressiva*[30]. In a footnote to the original paper, he stated that the term 'encephalitis' was used here in a broad sense, meaning disease of the brain and not brain inflammation. The illness usually began between the ages of 50 and 65, with slow progression of mental deterioration, often extending over 10 years; other symptoms of cerebral arteriosclerosis may appear during its course.

Olszewski[31] reviewed the literature on 'Binswanger's disease', noting that it was Alzheimer who had attached Binswanger's name to this variety of cerebral arteriosclerosis in 1902[32]. According to Olszewski, a more detailed description was promised by Binswanger, but never appeared[33]. In the almost 70 years between Binswanger's original description and this review, only about 30 cases were reported in the scientific literature, with Olszewski adding two more. But since the advent of modern brain imaging techniques in the 1970s, many papers have been published, mainly in neurological and radiological journals, reporting hundreds of cases. Some of these give the impression that the understanding of Binswanger's disease has changed with the introduction of new terminology. For instance, in 1972, De Reuck & Schaumburg published a paper entitled 'Periventricular atherosclerotic leukoencephalopathy'[34]. In 1986, Lotz *et al* reviewed subcortical arteriosclerotic encephalopathy, correlating computerised tomography (CT) and pathological findings; their references showed the name of Binswanger appearing in the title of 11 papers published between 1973 and 1984[35]. In 1987, Hachinski *et al* suggested the general term 'leuco-araiosis' to describe the common denominator of white matter changes in demented individuals, which consisted of decreased density seen on CT scans or a change in the bound hydrogen signal on magnetic resonance imaging (MRI); 'leuco-araiosis' referred to diminution of the density of representation of the white matter[36]. In 1988 the condition was further refined by Drayer, who introduced the term 'Binswanger microangiopathic leukoencephalopathy' to describe the spectra of abnormalities of the vascular supply to the cerebral white matter and basal ganglia[37].

Most of these authors stressed the facts that Binswanger's disease, however defined, was difficult to diagnose clinically, and that the localisation of the vascular disorders had changed from that in Binswanger's own cases, which showed predominant involvement in the temporo-occipital area, to the findings from brain imaging of predominant involvement in the periventricular area near the frontal horn. Before the currently widely used term 'multi-infarct dementia' was introduced in 1974[38] (see chapter in this book), the usual clinical diagnosis of patients thus afflicted was 'psychosis with cerebral arteriosclerosis'; Binswanger's disease was therefore, and still is to be regarded as a subtype of this condition.

Otto Binswanger (1852-1929)
Born in Munsterlingen on the Swiss shores of Lake Constance, Binswanger was the son of the director of the Kantonspital—a former Benedictine monastery which had been converted into a psychiatric hospital. Binswanger followed in his father's footsteps, in that having completed his undergraduate and postgraduate medical studies, he was appointed assistant physician at the provincial psychiatric hospital in Göttingen, North Germany in 1877. After short assignments in Breslau and Berlin, he settled down in Jena, where he spent the next 37 years, the last 28 as professor of psychiatry at the University. It was there that he wrote his only paper on the disease that carries his name. In 1919, Binswanger retired to Kreuzlingen, close to where he was born. There, he worked side by side with his nephew Ludwig, who eventually became more famous than Otto, as one of the pioneers of existential analysis. Otto remained professionally active almost until his death at the age of 76, having published more than 100 papers on a variety of psychiatric topics. With Siemerling, he also edited a popular textbook of psychiatry, and was much in demand as a lecturer. Although he had offers from several other universities, he remained faithful to his own University of Jena, where he was Rector twice[33].

Wilson's Disease
In 1912, Kinnier Wilson published a monograph entitled 'Progressive lenticular degeneration: a familial disease associated with cirrhosis of the liver'[39]. Others had made clinical reports of this disease, but it was Wilson who detected the association between liver disease and the degeneration of the lenticular nuclei. His work was based on four personal cases, together with notes on the unpublished cases of others. The disease is now known to be a rare, recessively inherited condition, in which an error of copper metabolism leads to the deposition of the metal in the brain and liver. The type of dementia associated with the disease was characterised by slowness of mental powers, listlessness, emotionalism, and childishness; Wilson recognised that these mental changes were different from those seen

in dementia paralytica, but similar to the ones seen in Huntington's chorea.

S. A. Kinnier Wilson (1878-1937)

Born in Cedarville, New Jersey, Wilson moved with his family to Scotland. Having obtained MA, MB, and MSc degrees at Edinburgh University, he continued his studies in Paris and Leipzig, before being appointed to the staff of the National Hospital, Queen Square, London, where he remained for 33 years, and was a colleague of the famous neurologists Gowers and Hughlings Jackson. Wilson's work on hepato-lenticular degeneration, for which he became famous early in his professional career, was published in 1912 and gained him the degree of MD with gold medal. Wilson was an excellent teacher of neurology; his lectures had a dramatic and compelling quality and did much to enhance Queen Square as a teaching centre. In 1920, he founded the *Journal of Neurology & Psychopathology*. He died at the age of 58, unfortunately before he had quite completed his textbook of neurology[40].

Brain tumours

It is not possible to pinpoint the occurrence of subcortical dementia in the symptomatology of brain tumours, because of the great variability in the types and the sites of these lesions, as well as the secondary symptoms due to increased intracranial pressure. However, two publications in which dementia of the subcortical type was alluded to in the description of certain kinds of neoplasms deserve mention. In their 1938 report on tumours of the thalamus, Smyth & Stern referred to a paper by Pfeifer in 1910 on psychic disturbances occurring in patients with brain tumours[41]. They themselves described six cases (five gliomas and one sarcoma), four of which presented with early dementia and originated in the thalamus, whereas in the other two, the tumour arose in the neighbouring internal capsule and dementia occurred late in the course of the disease.

In 1931, a discussion was held at the Royal Society of Medicine in London on the mental symptoms associated with cerebral tumours; Kinnier Wilson was then President of the Section of Psychiatry[42]. Of the eight other participants three were famous neurologists—Gordon Holmes, Russell Brain, and Charles Symonds—and one a distinguished psychiatrist—Edward Mapother. Wilson concluded the discussion by expressing the consensus of the group that 'the localising value of mental symptoms in cases of cerebral tumour was practically nil'.

Hallervorden-Spatz Disease

In 1922, Hallervorden & Spatz reported an unusual extrapyramidal syndrome that appeared in five out of 12 siblings of an unfortunate family. The disorder began between the ages of seven and nine, and progressed to death between 16 and 27 years. The lesions were in the globus pallidus and substantia nigra. Two variants of this condition were later reported, one starting in the second year of life, the other becoming manifest in middle age; dementia is a prominent feature[43].

Postencephalitic Parkinsonism

Encephalitis lethargica became a well known inflammatory disease, presumably of viral origin, when it reached epidemic proportions from 1919 to 1926. Motor disturbances resembling Parkinsonism sometimes appeared soon after the acute phase had subsided, but at other times several years later. Bebb in 1925 was one of the first to describe memory disturbances as part of the clinical picture of postencephalitic Parkinsonism; these were apparently not cortical in origin, but due to lesions in the substantia nigra and other basal nuclei[44].

Idiopathic Calcification of the Basal Ganglia

In 1935, Kasanin & Crank reported a case of extensive calcification of the brain[45]; other authors later described similar cases, involving primarily the basal ganglia, and manifesting progressive Parkinsonism, choreo-athetosis, and dementia of the subcortical type. Early-onset cases (age-range 20 to 40 years) may present with schizophrenia-like symptoms, whereas later-onset cases (age-range 40 to 60 years) usually show dementia and movement disorders at first.

Thalamic dementia

In 1939 Stern[46] and in 1942 Grunthal[47] published case reports of bilaterally symmetrical atropic lesions of the thalamus; the patients had profound dementia. Grunthal's patient had choreiform movements, and at autopsy showed atrophy of the red nucleus as well as of the thalamic nuclei.

Lacunar state

Although this condition is a variety of vascular dementia similar to Binswanger's disease, it may be briefly mentioned here because the lesions are mainly subcortical. Lacunes are small ischaemic infarcts most commonly located in the basal ganglia, thalamus, and internal capsule; the aetiology is thrombotic or embolic. Davison and Brill in 1939 were among the first to describe these lesions, as part of their study of chronic hypertensive encephalopathy[48].

Parkinson-dementia complex of Guam

One of the most unusual conditions was first described by Hierano et al in 1961[49]: on the island of Guam in the Western Pacific:

10% of adult deaths result from amyotrophic lateral sclerosis, and 7% are the consequence of a Parkinson-dementia complex. The two conditions appear to be variants of a single disease process. Dementia occurs early, with Parkinsonism and other neurological signs developing later in the clinical course. The average age of onset is 50 years, with a range from 32 to 77 years; death occurs in four to five years. It is not known if the aetiology is primarily hereditary or environmental.

Spinocerebellar degenerations

In 1954, Greenfield wrote a classical monograph on the spino-cerebellar degenerations[50], which are a heterogeneous group of disorders affecting principally the hindbrain and the spinal cord, but also often extending upwards into the basal nuclei, and thereby producing dementias of the subcortical type. One of the earliest papers was that of Neff, who in 1894 reported on 13 cases of ataxia in adults with hereditary history. Cummings & Benson[51] mention at least 25 other papers published by various authors between 1902 and 1982 on cerebellar and olivopontocerebellar degenerations with the characteristics of subcortical dementia.

Progressive supranuclear palsy

In 1963, Richardson *et al* drew attention to a very unusual extra-pyramidal syndrome characterised by a combination of neuro-ophthalmic symptoms (pseudobulbar palsy with loss of volitional downward gaze), bradykinesia, mask-like facies, rigidity of the neck and trunk with hyper-erect posture, and either early or late dementia[52]. Similar cases had been described before[53], but these authors established the condition as a clear nosological entity[54].

In progressive supranuclear palsy, the atrophic lesions, which include the presence of neurofibrillary tangles, are located in the subthalamic nucleus, substantia nigra, globus pallidus, superior colliculus, peri-aqueductal grey matter, and dentate nucleus of the cerebellum. The oculomotor, trochlear, and abducens nuclei are also affected, but the cortex is normal. The type of dementia seen was different from the typical cortical dementias, and in 1974, it led Albert *et al* to revive the concept of subcortical dementia[55].

Progressive subcortical gliosis

In 1967, Neumann & Cohn reported four cases of an insidious progressive dementia where the most prominent histological feature was pronounced subcortical gliosis, without severe involvement of the cortex[56]. The basal ganglia, thalamus, brain stem nuclei, and ventral horns of the spinal cord were also affected; the gliosis appeared to be the primary pathology. These authors compared the condition with Alzheimer's and Pick's disease because the clinical features were quite similar; however, histopathological examination revealed that there was absence of argyrophilic plaques and neurofibrillary changes, and that the cortical nerve cell loss was relatively mild.

Past, present and future

In the history of the concept of 'subcortical dementia', certain trends can be discerned: the gradual evolution and increasing sophistication of the way in which different conditions are described in the literature; the various technical advances, from at first purely clinical observations, via pathological descriptions of autopsy material, improved staining techniques for differentiating histological changes, the early development of electroencephalography and pneumoencephalography, to the modern brain imaging techniques; as well as changing patterns in the practice of medicine, from general practice (Parkinson, Huntington) to neuropsychiatry (Binswanger, Wilson), and more recently to much greater contributions by neurologists and radiologists. Modern psychiatrists have not been particularly active in this area; the closest they have come is their concern with tardive dyskinesia, which does not apparently produce any signs of dementia—subcortical or cortical.

We still know relatively little about the aetiology of most of the dementias, nor are there curative treatments for them, but no matter how mysterious and bizarre many of these conditions appear to be, some of them have a particular fascination. The fact that even today, a number of them are best known by their eponyms adds to their interest. Huntington's chorea is perhaps the most prominent of this group of diseases, as it is the only one that has a persistently clear-cut hereditary basis, presents such a striking clinical picture, and is so widespread. Behind the apparent, often rather dry objectivity of the descriptions of the dementias in the scientific literature, there is a vast amount of suffering and distress in the afflicted patients and their families, for whom we can still offer little but our sympathy and support. At the same time, the history of subcortical dementia has shown how much can be accomplished by various professionals in the search for understanding how the different parts of the central nervous system function in relation to one another in health and in disease. Further generations of neurologists, psychologists, psychiatrists, and research workers of many backgrounds must continue to collaborate closely in seeking a still better understanding and much more successful methods of treatment of these diseases.

Chapter 7

Other Forms of Dementia

G. E. Berrios

By the end of the nineteenth century, three general forms of dementia were recognised: senile, arteriosclerotic, and subcortical. These groupings, however, were not exhaustive and a number of clinical states resembling dementia did not fit well into them. Some of these, such as general paralysis of the insane, dementia praecox, and melancholia attonita had been known for a long time, others such as the cognitive failure caused by alcoholism, epilepsy, brain damage, and intoxication with lead were becoming fashionable, while yet others, such as pseudo-dementia and Creutzfeldt-Jakob disease were about to be discovered. Alienists solved this problem of classification in several ways. Firstly, the forms of dementia already well known continued in use, except for dementia praecox and melancholia attonita, which were reclassified as 'schizophrenia' and 'stupor' respectively. Secondly, the 'new' forms of dementia were named after either their putative cause or their discoverer, e.g. dementia dialytica and Creutzfeld-Jakob disease. Finally, notions such as 'reversible dementia' and 'pseudo-dementia' were created to include a number of ambiguous clinical states. The conceptual issues generated by these temporary solutions are still with us today; this chapter deals with their history.

General paralysis of the insane
In 1821, ALJ Bayle published under the name *arachnitis chronique*[1] a partial description of what has since been known as 'general paralysis of the insane'. It has been claimed that this 'new phenomenon' resulted from 'a mutation in the syphilitic virus towards the end of the eighteenth century' (p623)[2] and that its discovery reinforced the belief of alienists in the anatomo-clinical view of mental disease, but that this 'proved a step backward for the general psychopathology of the severe neuroses and psychoses' (p399)[3]. Another view is that general paralysis 'became the model of a psychiatry conceived exclusively as a natural science' (p224)[4]. However, the concept was never very clear-cut. It took the best part of 30 years for general paralysis to gain acceptance as a 'separate' disease, and far from making alienists more organically orientated, this embroiled them in all manner of psychological and philosophical issues such as the mind body-problem, brain localisation, and psychological causation[4,5].

Bayle's 'discovery' of general paralysis was a challenge to the 'cross-sectional' view of disease, and indeed of medical diagnosis in general which looked at the patient at one point in time[6]. He believed that clinical conditions needed a longitudinal redefinition, in terms of temporal patterns of symptoms, which would guarantee their continuity as entities with an anatomical basis. As Bercherie put it: 'for the first time in the history of psychiatry there was a morbid entity which presented itself as a sequential process unfolding itself into successive clinical syndromes' (p75)[7].

By the middle of the nineteenth century, though, no agreement had yet been reached as to how symptoms were caused in the *periencephalite chronique diffuse* that general paralysis was then named[8]. Three clinical subtypes were recognised: manic-ambitious, melancholic-hypochondriac, and dementia. According to the 'unitary view', all three constituted stages of a single disease[1], the order of their appearance depending on the progress of the cerebral lesions. Baillarger, on the other hand, sponsored the 'dualist' view that 'paralytic insanity and paralytic dementia are different conditions'[8]. This debate, however, had less to do with the nature of the brain lesions than with their capacity to generate mental symptoms: how could the 'typical' content of paralytic delusions (grandiosity) and the general demeanour of the paralytic patient be explained? Baillarger believed that chronic periencephalitis could only account for motor signs; since the symptoms might also be found in subjects without brain lesions—'they must have a different origin' (p389)[8]. This absence of any link between the lesion and the symptom would explain why patients might recover.

The idea that general paralysis was related to syphilis had been discussed since the work of Fournier in 1875[9]. However, there was resistance to the view that the similar clinical states seen in many syphilitic patients were actual instances of Bayle's disease, and the term 'pseudo-general paralysis' was coined to refer both to its delusional (grandiose) form and to one with dementia[10]. But if nineteenth-century alienists were indeed organic in approach, why did they not fully accept the suggestion of a syphilitic aetiology?

There is surprisingly little evidence that alienists then considered general paralysis a 'paradigm-disease', i.e. as the aetiological and clinical model for all other mental diseases. The new illness, though, actually created more problems than it solved[11]: its definition included a great variety of symptoms, and because it was widely believed that affective symptoms had to be an early manifestation, patients with what would now be considered typical manic-depressive illness were diagnosed as suffering from general paralysis. In 1889, however, Baillarger questioned the clinical boundaries of GPI, concluding that patients might exhibit all its symptoms without in fact suffering from it, and that those with 'pseudo-general paralysis' might improve[10]. Even more challenging was the decision of the

Berlin meeting of 1883 that the 'disease', after all, had no 'typical' anatomo-pathology[12], as had previously been claimed, since a number of the changes reported by Bayle were due to *post-mortem* brain lysis.

Dementia praecox becomes schizophrenia

Morel coined the term *démence précoce* to refer to a state of dementia occurring during adolescence or soon after[13], and Kraepelin borrowed it to name the composite disease[14] that was soon after to be further renamed 'schizophrenia' by Bleuler[15]. Later, Kurt Schneider suggested a set of 'empirical' diagnostic criteria to define the new disease[16], which have become part of current clinical practice. The work of these four men thus provides the axis for all histories of schizophrenia[17-19], but it remains uncertain whether this is the history of a term, a concept, a behavioural repertoire, or of all three. Can it be assumed that the disease 'existed' throughout (or even before) the nineteenth century? The lack of clear reports before 1850[20-23] has been interpreted as meaning that the disease did not exist then[24]; that 'schizophrenia' has a social origin, and that the 'cases' seen today might just be sequelae of encephalitic diseases, for instance[25]. However, the absence of such reports does not mean that the illness did not exist—it may simply be that it was not recognised or described then. Neither can any conclusion be drawn about its aetiology, even if the illness had emerged *de novo* during this period, since it could have resulted from a number of factors such as a genetic mutation or a new infection.

Did Morel, then, describe schizophrenia for the first time? The conventional account is that he coined the term *démence précoce* to describe a disease causing severe cognitive impairment and psychosocial incompetence in young people[7], though both the English apothecary Hallam[26] and Pinel[27] are said to have identified similar clinical states earlier, using different names for them. Morel's term appeared for the first time in 1852, applied to the same clinical state that Georget and others had until then called 'stupidity'—a collection of syndromes whose only common denominator was non-responsiveness. Morel[13] actually reported the case of a young man who, after a religious phase and one of deluded and hallucinatory excitement, developed generalised muscular contractions. The patient then went into a six-months' stupor, during which he maintained awkward bodily positions, would not answer questions, and was incontinent. After months more, he improved somewhat, but remained lacking in initiative and showed automatic behaviour. It is tempting to re-diagnose this case as one of catatonic schizophrenia[28], but all one can conclude is that these clinical states were already in existence, and that they were perceived through very different diagnostic filters. Kahlbaum[29] wrote his book on 'catatonia' to re-assess 'stupidity', emphasising the motor aspects of the disorder. Kraepelin's contribution was to suggest that it should be brought together with dementia paranoides, simplex, and hebephrenia under the umbrella of a putative disease that was based on a bad prognosis and common anatomo-pathology[14].

Dementia praecox became 'schizophrenia' in a book published by Bleuler in 1911[15]; the main ideas derived from a collective intellectual effort in the Burghölzli Hospital, Zürich[19], which is why Jung's monograph (1907) on the 'Psychology of dementia praecox'[30] contains very similar concepts. Bleuler, was one of the first asylum psychiatrists to apply Freudian concepts to the psychoses, but his notion of schizophrenia was also shaped by Kraepelin's definition, associationism, faculty psychology, the psychodynamic *Zeitgeist*, his ample clinical experience, and probably the nationalistic redefinition of Swiss *vis-à-vis* German psychiatry. He justified his preference for the word schizophrenia (which he had used for the first time in 1908) by saying that the old term had become too fatalistic and was often taken literally to mean dementia affecting the young[19]. But as is often the case, a change in name led to a change in the controlling metaphor: the notion of 'splitting' ('*Spaltung*'), the basis of his new diagnostic term, became influential during this period[31].

Characteristically, instead of producing a speculative pathophysiology of dementia praecox, Kraepelin offered a description, a natural history, and a prognosis[32]. Around the beginning of this century, explanations of symptoms as symbolic representations of processes occurring beyond awareness became popular, so that those of schizophrenia, including the motor and cognitive symptoms, were 'psychologised'. For example, stereotypies and echo phenomena were no longer considered as disorders of the motor system, but of the will[33]. Bleuler's new conception of the disease offered the psychiatric community a compromise between remaining loyal to the old neuropsychiatry and adopting psychodynamic ideas: the symptoms became 'understandable', and the result was to conjure the dementia out of existence[19]. It remained there until after the second World War, when once again the defect state began to be interpreted in organic terms[34].

Pseudo-dementia and vesanic dementia
Though there is a growing interest in pseudodementia[35-38], neither the term, the concept, nor the issues they raise are new. As during the late nineteenth century, questions are now asked as to whether the 'dementia' of pseudodementia is real or just a bad copy (a phenocopy)[38]. This concept was created as a solution to the problem of reversibility and was also discussed under the name of *démence melancolique*[39]. To bring under this heading the Ganser syndrome and other prison psychoses is likely to confuse the issue, though, since their original description did not include 'dementia' amongst the symptoms. Nor was it meant to deal with the issue of irreversibility:

indeed, Ganser's descriptions[40] were associated with the concept of hysterical twilight state, and Sommer's prison psychoses[41] with that of paranoid disease.

One of the earliest writers to study the condition was Mairet at Montpellier in 1883[39]. Before this time, cases of dementia that improved had usually been explained as being 'vesanic' dementia, i.e. caused by a functional psychosis[42]. However, Mairet challenged this compromise with cases which were reversible but showed brain changes. His finding that melancholic patients with cognitive impairment had changes in the temporal lobe led him to hypothesise that this area might be related to feelings of sadness, and that the nihilistic delusions were secondary, due to diffuse spread of the lesion to the cortex. Mairet's cases (some of which would now be called Cotard's syndrome)[43] became retarded, refused food, and ended up in states of stupor; many went on to die from metabolic or infectious complications. They represent what was eventually to be called 'depressive pseudodementia'. Mairet was not trying to create yet another disease, but to identify lesions that might account for the mood disorder, analyse melancholic delusions into their component parts, and relate each to a different brain site. He did not believe that the form of the delusion was related to the lesion, but that lesions in certain sites 'give rise to emotional changes in the direction of sadness'[39].

The other great contributor was George Dumas, whose thesis[44] was to have great impact on both French and German thinking in this field. He concluded that it was 'mental fatigue that explained the psychological poverty and monotony of melancholic depressions' and that the problem was not 'an absence but a stagnation of ideas'[44]. He also offered probably the first cognitive model of depression.

The term pseudodementia, though had started in a different intellectual and clinical tradition[38]. Wernicke used it first to refer to 'a chronic hysterical state mimicking mental weakness'[45]— almost tantamount to the Ganser syndrome. It did not come into general use then, but was resuscitated in the 1950s[46,47]. It has since acquired at least three meanings: a reversible cognitive impairment in psychosis, a copy or parody of such impairment, and the temporary impairment resulting from delirium[38]. Pseudodementia still has a role to play in current psychiatric practice—to draw attention to states of reversible cognitive incompetence which are not due to failure of performance[38].

Presbyophrenia and confabulation

The word 'presbyophrenia' was coined by Kahlbaum[48] for a subtype of the paraphrenias, i.e. forms of insanity occurring during periods of biological change, the *hebetica* type affecting adolescents, and the *senilis* the elderly. Presbyophrenia, the main type of paraphrenia senilis, described a state of disorientation, amnesia, delusional misidentification, and confabulation. Kahlbaum's innovative taxonomy, unnoticed for 40 years, emerged only in the later work of Kraepelin[32], Fischer[49], and Wernicke[50].

Wernicke's classification was based on consciousness being associated with three categories of objects: the outside world, the body, and the self, their individual impairment giving rise to different psychoses[50]. The first of these included delirium tremens, Korsakoff's psychosis, presbyophrenia, acute and chronic hallucinoses, and pathological drunkenness. Amongst the features of presbyophrenia, Wernicke included confabulations, disorientation, hyperactivity, euphoria, and a fluctuating course. An acute form was said to resolve without trace, while the chronic merged into senile dementia, but he did not make clear whether he considered presbyophrenia a separate disease[51,52].

By 1906, Rouby[53] had identified one type of presbyophrenia as a form of senile dementia which included impairment of memory, disorientation, confabulation, misidentification, cognitive impairment, pathological euphoria, delusions, hallucinations, agitation, nightmares, and occasionally somnolence. He concluded that presbyophrenia was a final common pathway for cases suffering from Korsakoff's psychosis, senile dementia, or acute confusion. Two prominent French psychiatrists of the first half of this century, Truelle & Bessière[54], however, suggested that it might be the expression of a toxic state caused by liver or kidney failure. It was not always easy, though, to distinguish the elevated mood of the presbyophrenic from the hypomanic form of general paralysis, and confusional states were also considered as both a possible mechanism and a differential diagnosis. The French view was that presbyophrenia was characterised by three fundamental symptoms: confabulation, disorientation, and amnesia for recent events, but this blurred the boundaries between it and Korsakoff's psychosis even further[55].

Kraepelin[56] included presbyophrenia in the senile and presenile insanities, describing it as a form of senile dementia, to be differentiated from Korsakoff's psychosis: presbyophrenic patients were older, showed no symptoms of polyneuritis, had no history of alcoholism, and exhibited more hyperactivity and elevated mood. Ziehen[57] wrote that 'the marked memory impairment contrasts with the relative sparing of thinking', while in 1907, Oskar Fischer described disseminated cerebral lesions, which he believed to be the essential anatomical substratum[49].

Views on presbyophrenia arrived in North America in 1913 in a translation of a paper by Nouet[58,59], who defended the view that it was a variety of senile dementia. A similar view was taken by Barret who considered presbyophrenia the 'best characterised of the senile mental disorders', and remarked on the 'striking disproportion between the ability of the patient to carry out an orderly conversation and yet have a profound disturbance of memory and orientation'. However, Bleuler[45] complained that its meaning varied 'according to the author and even in the same author at different times'. Wollenberg considered presbyophrenia a special form of senile psychosis and remarked upon the relative preservation of judgment and social graces shown by these patients[60].

During the 1930s, two new hypotheses emerged. Boestroem[61] concluded on phenomenological grounds that presbyophrenia could be identified with mania; he suggested that cerebral arteriosclerosis provided a general pathogenic factor, the specific factor being a cyclothymic pre-morbid personality. Lafora[62] emphasised the role of cerebrovascular pathology, and claimed that disinhibition and presbyophrenic behaviour were caused by a combination of senile and atherosclerotic changes. Burger-Pritz and Jacob[63], however, questioned whether cyclothymic features were a necessary pre-condition; they pointed out a double dissociation—that the syndrome was seen in patients without cyclothymia, and that hypomanic individuals did not necessarily develop presbyophrenia. In 1948, Bessière[64] claimed that presbyophrenia was a recognisable syndrome but not a separate disease—a mixture of confusion, confabulation, and dementia found in association with various disorders—senile dementia, brain tumours, traumatic psychoses, and confusional states. Henri Ey[65,66] supported this view and suggested that con-fabulation in the presbyophrenic was a 'compensatory' act, resulting from the utilisation of old information to fill current memory gaps; misidentifications and reduplicative paramnesias (distortion of memory involving geographical locations) were but forms of the same syndrome.

In spite of these efforts, presbyophrenia soon became forgotten, leaving three issues unresolved[51,52]. These were: firstly, the role played by cyclothymic personality or concomitant manic illness in the clinical profile of dementia; secondly, the role of delirium, 'oneiric' or dreamy states, confusion, and toxic states in the expression of the condition; and, thirdly, the pathogenic function of cerebrovascular disease, with the particular involvement of the frontal and occipital lobes. Of all the symptoms of presbyophrenia, confabulation has been the most striking and mysterious; it remains the linking concept with Korsakoff's psychosis, senile and multi-infarct dementia, hypomania, and cortical blindness[67]. In the latter, denial of illness is a form of confabulation; this behaviour may be mediated by a lesion resulting from an occlusion of the posterior cerebral artery, with involvement of occipital cortex and hippocampal-mamillary-thalamic-cingulate circuit (the latter causing a Korsakoff-like state)[68]. However, non-specific toxic-confusional states may be sufficient to trigger episodic confabulatory behaviour in individuals suffering from a loss of afferent stimuli[69].

Creutzfeldt–Jakob disease

The condition nowadays called Creutzfeldt–Jakob disease (CJD)[70] was described by two students of Alzheimer during the 1920s, though as is often the case with complex and uncommon conditions, the first identification remains uncertain. However, the fact that what used to be called Jakob-Creutzeldt disease has been changed to this form suggests that HG Creutzfeldt was the pioneer. ICD-10 defines the disease as: 'a progressive dementia with extensive neurological signs, due to specific neuropathological changes (subacute spongiform encephalopathy) which are presumed to be caused by a transmissible agent. Onset is usually in middle or later life . . . there is usually a progressive spastic paralysis of the limbs, accompanied by extrapyramidal signs with tremor, rigidity, and choreoathetoid movements. Other variants may include ataxia, visual failure, or muscle fibrillation and atrophy of the upper motor neuron type. The triad consists of rapidly progressive devastating dementia, pyramidal and extrapyramidal disease with myoclonus, and characteristic triphasic electroencephalogram is thought to be highly suggestive of the disease'.

In 1920, Creutzfeldt[71] reported the case of Berta E a 23 year-old woman who had been admitted in 1913 to the Neurological Clinic of Breslau University; Alzheimer was already in Breslau then, but it is not known whether he ever saw this case. At 21, she seems to have had an anorexic episode, and when admitted a year earlier for a skin condition, she was noticed to have spastic legs, tremor, and 'hysterical' behaviour. Just before the neurological admission, her gait disturbance returned and she became unkempt, developing nihilistic delusions. On admission, she was emaciated and showed generalised muscle fibrillations, hypertonia, and a fever (39°). She was disorientated, deluded, perseverative, and oscillating between excitement and stupor. She then developed epileptic attacks, and eventually died in status epilepticus. No cause or precipitating factor could be elicited: her *post-mortem* revealed a 'non-inflammatory focal disintegration of cortical tissue showing also neuronophagia, glial and some vascular proliferation, and a marked fall-out of grey cells everywhere'. Creutzfeldt considered multiple sclerosis as a possible diagnosis, but drew no definite conclusion as to the nature of the disorder. In 1921, A Jakob[72] reported four cases of a disorder which he considered resembled an acute form of multiple sclerosis, and which he denominated 'spastic pseudosclerosis'. The first was a 51 year-old woman with stiff legs, dizziness, fatigue, and later depression, ataxia, rigidity, and confusion; death occurred after one year of illness. The fourth case was that of a 43 year-old man who drank heavily, and after sustaining a hip fracture was unable to work again. He complained of stiff legs, headaches, and sometime later developed evening delirium with paranoid features; he began to hear voices during the day and to have sudden attacks of excitement. Admitted to a mental hospital with diagnosis of catatonia, he was intermittently stuporous, grimaced, and when occasionally accessible, was disorientated and confabulating. He died during one of his episodes of severe confusion. In all these cases, Jakob found great loss of ganglion-cells, glial proliferation, and fatty degeneration, the part of the brain most affected being the anterior part of the striatum and thalami. Jakob stated that: 'there have been few cases like these in the literature. The nearest is that of Creutzfeldt'[72]; about the predominant cortical involvement in the latter's case, he wrote: 'the more widespread distribution in Creutzfeldt's case, in the presence of similar lesions and symptoms, should not be taken as an important difference'. However, Creutzfeldt is said to have disagreed with this statement[73].

From this period on, the disease, then called 'spastic pseudo-sclerosis of Jakob', became lost in the group of basal ganglia degenerative states. However, interest in Kuru by Gajdusek[74] and in scrapie by Headlow[75] later led to the realisation that, like the other two diseases, CJD might be caused by a transmissible agent. In the event, brain tissue from a British patient affected with CJD was sent by Daniel *et al* to Gajdusek and Gibbs in the USA, who successfully transmitted the disease to a chimpanzee[76].

Pick's disease and the frontal dementias

The history of the dementias believed to be related to changes in the frontal lobes reveals why 'frontal dementias' have become fashionable once again[77,78]. When Pick described the syndrome since named after him, he wanted to draw attention to a form of dementia which was based on a local atrophy affecting the temporal lobe (as opposed to a generalised defect, as Wernicke believed)[79], which showed a preponderant dysfunction of language and praxis, and was susceptible to diagnosis during life. Pick suggested that these lobar atrophies merely constituted a period in the evolution of the senile dementias. The historical shift whereby Pick's disease came to be related to the frontal lobes requires explanation.

In 1857, Louis Pierre Gratiolet[80] re-named the cerebral lobes according to the name of the overlying bone: the 'anterior' lobe becoming the frontal lobe, but he made no functional assumption as to the role of the 'anterior extremity of the cerebral hemisphere'. Phrenology[81] had already related the reflective and perceptive functions to the forehead, but these were only qualitatively defined. 'Modular' assumptions (i.e. that one specific function was localised in one site) concerning the frontal lobes started in the 1860s, after published reports of an association between dysfunctions of language and lesions of the frontal lobes[82,83]. Until the end of the century, this belief ran parallel to British views, as propounded by Hughlings Jackson, that the cerebral cortex, being a human acquisition, was the general seat of personality and mind[84]. In 1884, Meynert[85] also had stated that 'the frontal lobes reach a high state of development in man', although he still believed that psychiatric illnesses were diseases of the 'fore-brain' (by which he meant the 'prosencephalon' or human brain as a whole). However, Pick did not relate behavioural changes to the frontal lobes in his first paper—on a case of focal senile atrophy and aphasia in a man of 71[86], nor when reporting his second case[87], a woman of 59 with generalised cortical atrophy, particularly of the left hemisphere. It was only in the fourth case[88], that of a 60 year-old man, that he referred to bilateral frontal atrophy.

Which of these cases, therefore, should be considered as the first of Pick's disease? At the time, no one thought that Pick had described a new disease; Barrett[89] interpreted two of Pick's cases as atypical forms of Alzheimer's disease, and Ziehen[57] did not see anything special in them. During the same period, Liepmann, Stransky, and Spielmeyer had described similar cases with aphasia and circumscribed cerebral atrophy[90], which led Urechia and Mihalescu to name the syndrome 'Spielmeyer's disease'[79]. However, in two papers on 'Pick's disease', Carl Schneider[91,92] created the condition by suggesting that it evolved in three stages—the first with a disturbance of judgement and behaviour, the second with localised symptoms (e.g. speech), and the third with generalised dementia. He recognised rapid and slow forms, the former with akinetic and aphasic subtypes and a malignant course, while the latter was associated with predominance of plaques (probably indistinguishable from Alzheimer's disease).

There is little doubt that Schneider's publications led to the crystallisation of the new disease. In ICD-10, it is described as: 'progressive dementia, commencing in middle life (usually between 50 and 60 years), characterised by slowly progressing changes in character and social deterioration leading to impairment of intellect, memory and language functions, with apathy, euphoria and, occasionally, extrapyramidal phenomena. The neuropathological picture is one of selective atrophy of the frontal and temporal lobes but without the occurrence of neuritic plaques and neurofibrillary tangles in excess of what is seen in normal ageing. Early onset cases tend to exhibit a more malignant course. The social and behaviour manifestations often antedate frank memory impairment'.

Dementia associated with brain damage

By the beginning of the twentieth century, the separation between 'traumatic neurasthenia' and dementia had been fully achieved[57]. The former referred to states of irritability, headache, hysterical dissociation, etc. occurring either together with or separately from cognitive impairment, while the notion of 'cognitive dementia' referred to a syndrome occurring after a severe brain injury. Variables affecting the development of traumatic dementia had by then been identified: whether, for example, the injury was open or closed, and whether it affected the top or the base of the skull; the type of pre-morbid personality and a history of alcoholism or arteriosclerosis were also important indicators.

To reach this clinical definition of the condition, experience was needed of the correlation of behavioural and neuropathological changes at *post-mortem*. The belief that only 'molecular', i.e. neuro-chemical changes were a feature of this condition was replaced, at the turn of the century, by the view that small haemorrhages and tissue tearing were probably responsible for the memory damage. Marie[93], for example, noted that when the 'lesion is localised in the frontal lobes, there is rapid mental decline'. During the latter part of the nineteenth century, traumatic dementia was discussed in the context of epileptic dementia[42], since it was believed that falls and brain injury were one of the factors that led to the latter. Yet dementia following trauma can already be found as a diagnostic category as early as in the work of Willis and of Cullen, respectively a century and two centuries before (see chapter 1).

Chapter 8

Dementia in Shakespeare's King Lear

J. G. Howells

In recent times, *King Lear* has come to displace *Hamlet* in general regard as Shakespeare's greatest play, though the reason for this was first enunciated by Samuel Johnson[1], who said 'This drama is the mirror of life'. In *King Lear*, Shakespeare's portrayal of life is at its most realistic and dramatic. His concentrated representation of life at its most harsh, turbulent, and fearful produces an intensity of action which is almost unbearable. Many have been unable to see the play a second time: all the main characters die tragically and there is no happy ending. The mood is caught by Gloucester thus: 'love cools, friendship falls off, brothers divide. In cities, mutinies; in countries, discord; in palaces, treason; and the bond cracked, twixt son and father . . . son against father . . . father against child' (I ii 115).

King Lear, the noble but wayward sovereign, displays the composite of two clinical conditions—firstly, dementia resulting from old age, and secondly, emotional illness resulting from the anguish of filial ingratitude—each impinging on the other. His condition is worsened by exposure during his wanderings; then he responds to the therapy of sleep and the affectionate care of his reconciled daughter, but emotion kills him—he dies from a 'broken heart' after the loss of this daughter.

The play
A synopsis of the play was supplied by Charles and Mary Lamb[2] in their first successful work, *Tales from Shakespeare*. The main plot concerns King Lear and his family, while a sub-plot features a noble, the Duke of Gloucester, and his family. The plots run parallel, meet at points, and finally come together in a dramatic climax of homicide, suicide, and stressful death.

Lear, King of England, has three daughters: Goneril, wife of the Duke of Albany; Regan, wife of the Duke of Cornwall; and Cordelia, successfully wooed by the King of France. The Duke of Gloucester has two sons: Edmund, a bastard, and Edgar, a legitimate son. King Lear, now over 80 years of age, decides to partition his kingdom between his three daughters. Before doing so, he applies a test of their love of him. Goneril and Regan counterfeit their love and fool the old man into giving them portions of his kingdom. Cordelia, honestly, insists on sharing her love between her father and her would-be husband:

'When I shall wed, That lord whose hand must take my plight shall carry Half my love with him'. (I i 102)

Rash, impulsive, irascible, wrathful, arrogant, the King disinherits Cordelia and shares his kingdom equally between Goneril and Regan and their husbands. Dependent on his daughters, the King is soon to regret his decision; systematically, they try to deprive him of everything.

In a fit of desperation, unable to stand the filial ingratitude any longer, he and his Fool leave Regan's household, only to find themselves in a storm on an inhospitable heath. Here, joined by a faithful retainer, he meets a Bedlam beggar, Poor Tom. This is Edgar in disguise, fleeing from his father and brother Edmund, since Gloucester had been persuaded by Edmund that Edgar plotted against his life. Fearful of his own life, Edgar has taken the disguise of Poor Tom. 'My cue is villainous melancholy, with a sigh like Tom o' Bedlam' (I ii 144). Lear's emotional torment matches the natural storm: the King finds himself as neglected as 'he of the basest form', Poor Tom.

Cordelia hastens from France with an army to recover his lands for Lear; she finds her father in a pitiful state, but they are reconciled. Though the war goes badly for Cordelia's forces, Goneril, in a fit of jealousy, poisons Regan and then commits suicide. Gloucester has his eyes gouged out by his son Edmund, but Edmund himself is killed in a dual with Edgar. Cordelia, by Edmund's secret order, has already been hanged and her lifeless body is brought in to Lear. The shock kills him: he bequeaths his lands to Edgar and dies.

Source material
Probably the most important background material is that concerning King Leir in *Holinshed's Chronicles*[3], but this is a very brief account and contains only the bare bones of the material used by Shakespeare. He was also influenced by an earlier play, *The True Chronicle History of King Leir*, published in 1605. There are other such minor sources as *The Mirour for Magistrates* (1587), Warner's *Albions England* (1586), and Spenser's *The Faerie Queene* (1591-1596). However, none of these sources contain the sub-plot present in Shakespeare's *King Lear*. Furthermore, in none of the sources is madness made a central feature of the play, and in all there is a contrived happy ending. Shakespeare would doubtless have heard of the senility of Brian Annesley, a contemporary gentleman pensioner of Queen Elizabeth, and of the loving care given him by his youngest daughter, Cordell. Whatever ideas Shakespeare had from his source material, though, these were enormously extended in his own version of the play. The material is very much Shakespeare's.

Themes in the play
Shakespeare's aim is to produce drama—not for kings and queens, professors of literature or philosophy, but for the simple audience

of his day. In the play, he is forced to take account of: the demands of drama; the players available and their skills; the sensitivity and views of his audience; the sensitivities of the royalty and politicians of his time; the knowledge available then; his previous plays; and current events. There is no mention of madness in any of the original material; this is introduced for purposes of drama and to exaggerate the points that he wishes to make.

The play has a moral aspect, since it is concerned with the rehabilitation of a soul. The King is forced to face up to his own defects, as the result of being reduced to the level of the humblest. The forces of good tend towards victory, but there is no certainty. Unlike its source material, the play does not indulge in happy endings. Elements of power and lack of it, wealth and poverty, ambition and humility, love and hate, are all at work. The King's rehabilitation starts on the heath when, in modesty, he turns to the Fool and says 'In boy, go first'. He is reduced to a 'nothing'. The Fool can say to him 'I am a Fool, thou art nothing' (I iv 200). Gloucester goes through the same humbling experience and can choose aid to the King before life. Edgar, hardened by the test of life, moves through the play from dupe to philosopher.

The play is also an essay on psychopathology. Shakespeare has chosen to portray the effects of stress on people; the central person has senile decay. To bring out truth, events are dramatised in an exaggerated way. Driven on by emotion, human affairs end in homicide, suicide, war, cruelty, and death. The central character is so stressed by emotion that it ultimately kills him.

To a clinician, the play is an exercise in family psychiatry[4]. It is concerned with two interacting families, within which, due to past events, emotional attitudes of great potential damage emerge. In both families, though, the biggest stress factor is filial ingratitude. This strikes King Lear so severely that when he sees mad Tom, he believes that noone could be reduced to that state other than by filial ingratitude. Sibling rivalry ends in the death of the two sisters, Goneril and Regan; husbands are of less importance than ambition, and are fair game for murder, while lust oversteps the boundaries of marriage. Being concerned with its present, the play does not answer questions dependent on the past. Where does the psychopathology of Goneril and Regan come from? In contrast, why the benevolence of Cordelia from the same family? The importance of love within the family is rated more highly than power or position. Neugebauer[5] has convincingly demonstrated that within the knowledge of the time, medieval psychiatry was eminently practical and unspeculative. Thus, interpretation of the play's events responds best to the approach of experiential psychopathology[6].

Where Shakespeare garnered his knowledge of abnormal psychology is a matter for conjecture. He lived at a time before Harvey's discovery of the circulation when 'scientific medicine', with its emphasis on the physical, had not yet destroyed the notion of the interplay of mind and body, which fostered an integrated approach to man's ills. In Shakespeare, there is a correct balance of attention to body and mind, not because he had any special knowledge or insight, but because he reflected the attitude of his times. There is evidence to show that he knew Philip Roger, the apothecary of Stratford, while his son-in-law, John Hall[7,8], was the physician of Stratford. However, Shakespeare's chief source may have been the literature of his time, in view of his well recognised acquaintance with the first English text in psychiatry, Timothy Bright's *Treatise of Melancholy*[9]. Dover Wilson[10] has exhibited many close parallels of thought and phrase between Hamlet and that Treatise. It is even speculated that Shakespeare was employed by Vautrollier, the publisher, as a press reader when Bright's book was being printed.

There are many additional clinical points of interest in the play, for instance, frequent references to the effect of emotion on the heart. 'Heart break' is given as a cause of death, for instance, of Gloucester— 'But his flawed heart . . . Burst smilingly' (V iii 198). The heart was probably blamed at times when cerebral catastrophes might actually have been responsible: a number of small emotionally precipitated cerebral incidents, or one major one, can be a potent cause of dementia. There is a vivid account of simulated insanity by Edgar, who takes the role of a Bedlam beggar; Shakespeare uses him for dramatic effect and no doubt exaggerates the picture. Psychopaths are prominent in the form of Goneril, Regan, Edmund, and Oswald. Edgar inflicts a pseudo-suicide on his father, in the hope that his survival will shock him to recovery. If anyone wrongly regards a court Fool as mentally retarded, he will be corrected by the person of the Fool here—a prime depository of ability, good humour, and wisdom.

Dementia

'Senile melancholy'—wrote Esquirol in 1845[11]—'is a state in which the old man . . . isolates himself, becomes sad, uneasy, hard to please, avaricious, suspicious and egotistical; often unjust towards his friends, his own children and society at large.' Shakespeare supports this picture in King Lear. In addition to the 'enfeeblement of great age', he makes much of the excessive emotionality released by Lear's enfeeblement—the tendency to be 'rash' and the 'unruly waywardness':

> 'The best and soundest of his time hath been but rash; then must we look from his age to receive not alone the imperfections of long-engraffed condition, but therewithal the unruly waywardness that infirm and choleric years bring with them' (I i 297).

Dementia leads to loss of judgement and thus to rash decisions, such as Lear's banishment of his most affectionate daughter and his placing himself in the power of the two unscrupulous ones. This loss of judgement is also recognised:

'Oh, Lear, Lear, Lear!
Beat at this gate that let thy folly in
And thy dear judgement out!' (I iv 277).

One of the cardinal symptoms of dementia is the loss of memory, especially for recent events, and thus inability to recognise people. The King can take the Fool, Edgar, and Kent for high justices:

Lear: 'I'll see their trial first,
                   Bring in their evidence.
(To Edgar):   Thou robed man of justice,
                   take thy place.
(To the Fool):   And thou, his yoke-fellow of equity,
                   Bench by his side.
(To Kent):   You are o' th' commission,
                   Sit you too'. (III vi 35).

When at his most distracted, Lear takes Gloucester for Goneril:

'Ha! Goneril with a white beard!' (IV vi 97).

Lear himself can half-perceive his forgetfulness, and has a feeling that he should be able to recognise those about him and remember recent events, which escape him, like blurred images from a dream:

'I fear I am not in my perfect mind,
Methinks I should know you, and know this man;
Yet I am doubtful; for I am mainly ignorant
What place this is; and all the skill I have
Remembers not these garments; nor I know not
Where I did lodge last night' (IV vii 63).

At times he is disorientated: distracted, he calls for supper in the morning: 'We'll go to supper 'i the' morning' (III vi 83). His Fool responds: 'And I'll go to bed at noon' (III vi 84). In his first contact with Cordelia at Dover, he is still disorientated: 'Am I in France?' (IV vii 76).

Defect of memory and disorientation in time and place leads to confusion—well portrayed here. Lear's thoughts become incoherent. In his agitated mind, images come and go in quick succession with no link between them. He suffers from misinterpreted phenomena, imagining himself to be recruiting men for his army and offering enlisting money (press money). He comments on a man handling his bow as if he was employed to scare crows. Then he thinks he sees a mouse and wants to catch it with a piece of cheese. In the next instant, he grabs his gauntlet and offers to fight a giant, whilst calling for the foot soldiers with their brown painted halberds (brown bills). The arrows image returns to his mind, and he sees it flying like a bird to the centre of the target (the clout):

> 'There's your press money. That fellow handles his bow like a crowkeeper; draw me a clother's yard. Look, look, a mouse! Peace, peace; this piece of toasted cheese will do't. There's my gauntlet; I'll prove it on a giant. Bring up the brown bills. O, well flow, bird! i' the clout, i' the clout—hewgh!' (IV vi 87).

Distracted and rambling, Cordelia receives a report on Lear:

> 'Alack, 'tis he: why, he was met even now
> As mad as the vexed sea; singing aloud;
> Crowned with rank femiter and furrow-weeds,
> With hardocks, hemlock, nettles, cuckoo-flow'rs,
> Darnel, and all the idle weeds that grow
> In our sustaining corn.' (IV iv 1-6).

Yet, Lear has insight—early on, he fears that stress will lead to loss of control: 'O, let me not be mad, not mad, sweet heaven! Keep me in temper; I would not be mad!' (I v 46). As matters worsen, he is less sure of maintaining control: 'O Fool, I shall go mad' (II iv 285). He puts the thought of filial ingratitude out of his mind, to protect it: 'No more of that' (III iv 21). As he recovers, he develops more insight: 'I fear I am not in my perfect mind.' (IV vii 63).

Psychopathology with dementia

There is continued reference to 'mad' or 'madness' in the play and various of the principal characters claim to be mad, to be becoming mad, or recovering from madness. However, they are not claiming a psychotic state, but rather that they are anguished, agitated, crazed, and upset, due to some obvious stress. The overwhelming stress is one of filial ingratitude—both the main and sub-plots turn around it.

To Be Mad

Kent explodes when Lear makes a misjudgement: 'Be Kent unmannerly When Lear is mad' (I i 148). Kent, having become irate with the servant Oswald, is asked by Cornwall if he is upset: 'What, art thou mad, old fellow?' (II ii 87). Lear curbs his irritation when about to speak to son-in-law Cornwall, so as not to lose self-control: 'We are not ourselves When nature, being oppressed, commands to mind' (II iv 104).

Gloucester reflects on Lear's state of mind and says, 'I am almost mad myself'. He emphasises that this is because his own long loved son wishes to take Gloucester's life—'The grief has crazed my wits.' (III iv 169 174). Kent explains Lear's state to Gloucester: 'All the power of his wits have given way to his impatience (rage).' (III vi 5). The doctor, about to administer drugs for Lear's madness at Cordelia's request, tells what it is for—'will close the eye of anguish' (IV iv 14). Kent comments to Gloucester 'His wits begin t' unsettle' (III iv 164), and Gloucester replies, 'Canst thou blame him?', as he goes on to explain that both Lear's daughters seek his death.

Course of Lear's disorder

Lear's disturbance moves through a number of stages. His vulnerable personality is initially traumatised by filial ingratitude. In the second stage, the disturbance becomes more acute after his confrontation with Tom on the heath, but is limited in duration, lasting from his exposure on the heath until his daughter's French army reaches him. In the third stage, he recovers completely with the help of his daughter and physician; indeed, he becomes joyful and controlled. But all is lost by the final, unexpected, overwhelming trauma—Cordelia's death. This precipitates not a disturbance, but death.

Filial ingratitude

Lear is clear about the source of his upset in the first stage: 'How sharper than a serpent's tooth it is To have a thankless child.' (I iv 295). Then, as his rejection becomes more acute, Lear comments: 'My wits begin to turn.' (III ii 68). However, he identifies his situation: 'The tempest in my mind Doth from my senses take all feeling else, Save what beats there. Filial ingratitude' (III iv 13). He resolves 'to weep no more'.

Disillusionment

The second stage leads to a heightening of his disturbance. Confronted by Tom o' Bedlam, he sees how low he has fallen: 'They told me I was everything; tis a lie.' (IV vi 106). And there comes final disillusion: 'Is man no more than this?' (III iv 105). Even here, filial ingratitude obtrudes. He can think of no other cause for Tom o' Bedlam's trials than: 'What, has his daughters brought him to this pass?' (III iv 63).

Recovery

After the reconciliation with Cordelia comes the recovery; guilt is relieved—and this despite both being prisoners—'I'll kneel down and ask of thee forgiveness' (V iii 10).

The physician applies three elements in his treatment. In the first, he prescribes rest; one of the many 'simples' (drugs) available will induce Lear to sleep and give him respite from the anguish that wears him down:

'Our foster-nurse of nature is repose,
The which he lacks; that to provoke in him
Are many simples operative, whose power
Will close the eye of anguish'.

As he recovers, the doctor calls for music—music therapy: 'Louder the music there!' (IV vii 25). In Shakespeare plays, there are at least 12 further examples of music therapy[12].

Thirdly, the doctor gives the King new clothes: '. . . . in the heaviness of sleep We put fresh garments on him.' (II vii 22). This could not but bring fresh confidence in being clothed again in a manner befitting a King. It may also have been used as a way of breaking through his confusion by presenting a familiar object. This device was used by Hughlings Jackson[13] when confronted by a postman in a post-epileptic confusional state: he instructed that the patient be given his post bag.

After Lear's recovery, the doctor is anxious that there should be no dwelling on the past: 'it is danger To make him even o'er the time he has lost.' (IV vii 80). This recovery is so complete that he can kill Cordelia's hangman: 'I killed the slave that was a-hanging thee' (V iii 276).

Death

But Lear was too late; the man had done his work. The nature of Lear's death may have been foretold in the play; earlier, he is suddenly extremely angry at the ill-treatment of his servant, which reflected on his own status: 'O, how this mother swells up toward my heart!' (II iv 55). The mother refers to hysteria, which was believed to have its origin in the womb of woman. Shakespeare may have been aware of a book, *A Brief Discourse of a Disease called the Suffocation of the Mother* by Edward Jordan[14], which was published in 1603—the time usually given for Shakespeare's work on King Lear. Both then and now, hysterical symptoms are often confused with psychosomatic symptoms. His anger threatens a heart attack, with its symptom of suffocation. Finally, aware of his daughter's death, he suddenly calls as he suffocates: 'Pray you, undo this button. Thank you, sir.' (V iii 311). He expires in a psychogenic death.

For him this is a welcome release, as Kent says when he stops Edgar's efforts to revive him:

'. . . O, let him pass! He hates him
That would upon the rack of this tough world
Stretch him out longer' (V iii 315).

Conclusion

So the old king dies, killed not by his venerable age, but by an emotion—grief. Esquirol[11] would have listed it under the heading of 'Moral' i.e. emotional causes; he presents two tables, one of physical and one of 'moral' causes of dementia. The highest single aetiological factor in the list of physical causes is 'progress of age', a daunting symptom, with no remedy; his list of 'moral causes' in his analysis of 40 cases reads as follows:

Disappointed affection   5
Frights   7
Political shocks   8
Disappointed ambition   3
Want   5
Domestic trials   12

Lear suffered them all, including 'want', in his aimless wanderings. But like less exalted mortals, it was his 'domestic trials', the damaging family relationships more than any other single factor that affected him deeply enough to lead to his death.

Shakespeare's picture of dementia may have one weakness. Throughout his disturbance, the King is made to grow in moral stature—he has learnt through his disturbing experience or as Edgar puts it:

'O, matter (sense) and impertinency (nonsense) mixed!
Reason in madness!' (IV vi).

In fact, it is rare in dementia to learn at all.

Chapter 1
Introduction

1   McMenemey WH. Alois Alzheimer and his disease. In: Wolstenholme GEW, O'Connor M (eds). *Alzheimer's Disease & Related Conditions*. London: J & A Churchill, 1970: pp 5-9.

2   Dillman R. *Alzheimer's Disease. The Concept of Disease and the Construction of Medical Knowledge*. Amsterdam: Thesis Publishers, 1990.

3   Berrios GE. Non-cognitive symptoms and the diagnosis of dementia. *Br J Psychiatry* 1989; **154** (Suppl): 11-16.

4   Wragg RE, Jeste DV. Overview of depression and psychosis in Alzheimer's disease. *Am J Psychiatry* 1989; **146**: 577-87.

5   Blumer A. The history and use of the term dementia. *Am J Insanity* 1907; **43**: 337-47.

6   Guiraud P. Evolution de l'idée de démence. *Ann Médico-Psychol* 1943; **101**: 186-99.

7   Marie A. *La démence*. Paris: Doin, 1906.

8   Berrios GE. The nosology of the dementias: an overview. In: Pitt B (ed). *Dementia*. Edinburgh: Churchill Livingstone, 1987: pp 19-55.

9   Kowalewski PJ. Sur la curabilité de la démence. *Ann Médico-Psychol* 1886; **44**: 40-53.

10 Berrios GE & Hauser R. The early development of Kraepelin's ideas on classification: a conceptual history. *Psychol Med* 1988; **18**: 813-21.

11 Jaspers K. Die Methoden der Intelligenzprüfung und der Begriff der Demenz. *Zeitschrift für des gesamte Neurologie und Psychiatrie (Referate und Ergebnisse)* 1910; **1**: 402-54.

12 D'Allones GR. *L'affaiblissement intelectuel chez les déments. Etude clinique par la méthode d'observation expérimentale*. Thèsis de Medecine Mentale, Faculté de Paris, 1912.

13 Toulouse E, Mignard M. Comment caractériser et definir la démence. *Ann Médico-Psychol* 1914; **72**: 443-61.

14 Berrios GE. Memory and the cognitive paradigm of dementia during the 19th century: a conceptual history. In: Murray RN, Turner TH (eds). *Lectures on the History of Psychiatry*. London: Gaskell, 1990: pp 194-211.

15 Courbon, (D'Amiens). Intégrité de la mémoire et démence. *Rev Psychiatrie* 1912; **16**: 448-55.

16 Berrios GE. Pseudodementia or melancholic dementia: a nineteenth century view. *J Neurol Neurosurg Psychiatry* 1985; **48**: 393-400.

17 Marcé LV. Recherches cliniques et anatomo-pathologiques sur la démence senile et sur les différences qui la separent de la paralysie générale. *Gazette Médicale de Paris* 1863; **34**: 433-5; 467-9; 497-502; 631-2; 761-4; 797-8; 831-3; 855-8.

18 Puillet P, Morel L. De la méthode des connaissances usuelles dans l'étude des démences. *J Psychol Normale Pathol* 1913; **10**: 25-36; 111-33.
19 McGaffin CG. An anatomical analysis of seventy cases of senile dementia. *Am J Insanity* 1910; **61**: 649-56.
20 Treadway WL. The presenile psychoses. *J Nerv Ment Dis* 1913; **40**: 375-87.
21 Pickett W. Senile dementia: a clinical study of two hundred cases with particular regard to types of the disease. *J Nerv Ment Dis* 1904; **31**: 81-8.
22 Southard EE. Anatomical findings in 'senile dementia': a diagnostic study bearing especially on the group of cerebral atrophies. *Am J Insanity* 1910; **61**: 673-708.
23 Bolton JS. The histological basis of amentia and dementia. *Arch Neurol* 1903; **2**: 424-612.
24 Marinesco G. Mécanisme de la sénilité e et de la mort des cellules nerveuses. *Comptes Rendus Hebdomadaires des Seances de l'Academie des Sciences* 1900; **130**: 1136-9.
25 Parchappe M. *Traité Théoretique et Pratique de la Folie*. Paris: Béchet Jeune et Labé, 1841.
26 Wilks S. Clinical notes on atrophy of the brain. *J Ment Sci* 1865; **10**: 381-92.
27 Hughes A. *A History of Cytology*. London: Abelard-Schuman, 1959.
28 Foucault M. *Naissance de la Clinique*. Paris: Presses Universitaires de France, 1963.
29 Maulitz RC. *Morbid Appearances. The Anatomy of Pathology in the Early 19th Century*. Cambridge: Cambridge University Press, 1987.
30 DeFelipe J, Jones J & EG. *Cajal on the Cerebral Cortex. An Annotated Translation of the Complete Writings*. Oxford: Oxford University Press, 1988.
31 Conn HJ. *The History of Staining*. Geneva: Biological Stain Commission, 1933.
32 Moya G, (ed). *Nicolás Achúcarro*. Madrid: Taurus Ediciones, 1968.
33 Spielmeyer W. *Technik der mikroskopischen Untersuchung des Nervensystems*. Berlin: Springer, 1911.
34 Ramón y Cajal S. *Neuronismo o reticularismo?* Madrid: CSIC, 1952.
35 Clarke E, Jacyna E, Jacyna LS. *Nineteenth-Century Origins of Neuroscientific Concepts*. Berkeley: University of California Press, 1987.
36 Fuller SC. A study of the neurofibrils in dementia paralytica, dementia senilis, chronic alcoholism, cerebral lues and microcephalic idiocy. *Am J Insanity* 1907; **63**: 415-68.
37 Ramón y Cajal S. *Recuerdos de mi Vida: Historia de mi Labor Científica*. Madrid: Alianza Editorial, 1981.

38 Parrot J. Cerveau. VIII Ramolissement. In: Dechambre A and Lereboullet L (eds). *Dictionnaire Encyclopédique des Sciences Médicales*. Vol 14. Paris: Mason and Asselin, 1873: pp 400-31.

39 Beljahow S. Pathological changes in the brain in dementia senilis. (reported in *J Ment Sci* 1889; **35**: 261-2).

40 Simchowicz T. Histologische Studien uber die senile Demenz. *Histol histopathol Arb Grosshirnr* 1911; **4**: 267-444.

41 Simchowicz T. Sur la signification des plaques séniles et sur la formule sénile de l'ecorce cerebrale. *Rev Neurol* 1924; **31**: 221-7.

42 Black SA. Pseudopods and synapses: the amoeoid theories of neuronal mobility and the early formulation of the synapse concept, 1894-1900. *Bull Hist Med* 1981; **55**: 34-58.

43 Billings SM. Concepts of nerve fiber development 1839-1930. *J Hist Biol* 1971; **4**: 275-305.

44 Gombault T. La démence terminale dans la psychose. *Ann Médico-Psychol* 1900; **58**: 231-249.

45 Ziehen T. Les démences. In: Marie A (ed). *Traité International de Psychologie Pathologique*, Vol 2. Paris: Alcan, 1911: pp 280-312.

46 Cordeiro JC. Etats délirants du troisième age. *L'Encephale* 1973; **62**: 20-55.

47 Plum F. Dementia: an approaching epidemic. *Nature* 1979; **279**: 372-3.

48 American Psychiatric Association: *Diagnostic and Statistical Manual of Mental Disorders*, 3rd Edition, Revised. Washington, DC: American Psychiatric Association, 1987.

49 Molsa PK, Paljary L, Rinne JO *et al.* Validity of clinical diagnosis in dementia: a prospective clinicopathological study. *J Neurol Neurosurg Psychiatry* 1985; **48**: 1085-90.

50 Wade JP, Mirsden TR, Hachinski VC *et al.* The clinical diagnosis of Alzheimer's disease. *Arch Neurol* 1987; **44**: 24-9.

51 Rocca WA, Amaducci L. The familial aggregation of Alzheimer's disease: An epidemiological review. *Psych Devel* 1988; **1**: 23-36.

52 Bondareff W. Age and Alzheimer's disease. *Lancet* 1983; **i**: 1447.

53 ICD-10 *1990 Draft of Chapter V. Mental and behavioural disorders*. Geneva: World Health Organisation, 1990.

54 Mayeux R, Stern Y, Spanton S. Heterogeneity in dementia of the Alzheimer type: evidence of subgroups. *Neurology* 1985; **35**: 453-61.

55 Brayne C, Calloway P. Normal ageing, impaired cognitive function, and senile dementia of the Alzheimer's type: a continuum? *Lancet* 1988; **i**: 1265-7.

56 Jorm AF. Subtypes of Alzheimer's dementia: a conceptual analysis and critical review. *Psychol Med* 1985; **15**: 543-53.

57 Maurer K, Riederer P, Beckmann H (eds). *Alzheimer's disease. Epidemiology, Neuropathology, Neurochemistry, and clinics*. Wien: Springer, 1990.

58 Harrison PJ. Pathogenesis of Alzheimer's disease—beyond the cholinergic hypothesis: a discussion paper. *J Roy Soc Med* 1986; **79**: 347- 52.

59 St George-Hyslop P, Tanzi RE, Polinski RG *et al.* The genetic defect causing familiar Alzheimer's disease maps on chromosome 21. *Science* 1987; **235**: 885-9.

60 de Leon MJ, George AE, Stylopoulos LA *et al.* Early marker for Alzheimer's disease: the atrophic hippocampus. *Lancet* 1989; **ii**, 672-3.

61 Duara R, Grady C, Haxby J *et al.*Positron emission tomography in Alzheimer's disease. *Neurology* 1986; **36**: 879-87.

62 Nebes RD. Semantic memory in Alzheimer's disease. *Psychol Bull* 1989; **106**: 377-94.

63 Amaducci L, Rocca WA, Schoenberg BS. Origin of the distinction between Alzheimer's disease and senile dementia. *Neurology* 1986; **36**: 1497-9.

64 Beach TG. The history of Alzheimer's disease. *J Hist Med Allied Sciences* 1987; **42**: 327-49.

65 Berrios GE. Alzheimer's disease: a conceptual history. *Int J Geriatric Psych* 1990; **5**: 355-65.

66 Hoff P, Hippius H. Alois Alzheimer 1864-1915. *Nervenarzt* 1989; **60**: 332-7.

67 Bick K, Amaducci L, Pepeu G. *The early story of Alzheimer's disease.* New York: Raven Press, 1987.

68 Bick K, Amaducci L (eds). *Alois Alzheimer & Gaetano Perusini: Alzheimer's first case rediscovered.* Padova: Liviana Press, 1989.

69 Förstl H, Levy RA. Alzheimer on certain peculiar diseases of old age. *History Psych* 1991; **2**: 71-101.

70 Hippius H. Aloys Alzheimer 14.06.1864-19.12.1915. In: Maurer K, Riederer P, Beckman H (eds). *Alzheimer's disease.* Wien: Springer, 1990: pp xiii-xix.

Chapter 2
Dementia Before the Twentieth Century

1 Lewis CT, Short C. *A Latin Dictionary.* Oxford: Clarendon Press, 1879: p 541.

2 Willis T. *Practice of Physick.* Translated by S. Pordage, London: T Dring, C Harper & J Leigh, 1684: pp 209-14. For a discussion of Willis's views see: Conry Y. Thomas Willis ou le premiere discours rationaliste en pathologie mentale. *L'Information Psychiatrique* 1982; **58**: 313-23; Cranefield PF. A seventeenth century view of mental deficiency and schizophrenia: Thomas Willis on 'stupidity or foolishness'. *Bull Hist Med* 1961; **35**: 291-316; Vinchon J, Vie J. Un maitre de la neuropsychiatrie au XVIII Siècle: Thomas Willis (1662-1675). *Ann Médico-Psychol* 1928; **86**: 109-44.

3   Blancard S. *The physical dictionary wherein the terms of anatomy, the names and causes of diseases, chirurgical instruments, and their use, are accurately described.* London: John and Benjamin Sprint, 1726.

4   Stephanus H. *Dictionarium medicum vel, expositiones vocum medicinatii, adverbum ex...*, (No place of publication) Huldrici Figgeri, 1564.

5   Kerckringii T. *Spicilegium anatomicum, continens observationum Anatomicarum rariorum centuriam unam.* Amsterdam: Andrea Frissii, 1670.

6   Baronio R. *A physical dictionary.* London: John Garfield, 1657.

7   Diderot & d'Alembert (eds). *Encyclopédie ou dictionnaire raisonné des sciences, des Arts et des métieres, par une societé de gens de lettres.* Paris: Briasson, David, Le Breton, Durand, Vol 4, 1754: pp 807-8.

8   Pinel Ph. *A Treatise on Insanity.* (translated by DD Davis). Sheffield: Cadell & Davies, 1806.

9   Cullen W. *Institutions de Médecine-Pratique*, traduites fur la quatrième & dernière Edition de l'Ouvrage anglois de M Cullen, par M Pinel, A Paris, Chez Pierre-J Duplain, 1785.

10 Sobrino. *Aumentado o Nuevo Diccionario de las lenguas española, francesa y latina*, León de Francia, JB Delamolliere, 1791.

11 Eloy NFI d'Aumont. In: *Dictionnaire historique de la médecine ancienne et moderne*, Vol 1. Paris: Mons, 1778: p 227. For a wider discussion of the medical writers of the French Encyclopaedia see: Astruc P. Les sciences médicales et leurs représentants dans l'Encyclopédie. *Revue Hist Sci* 1951; **4**: 359-68; Coleman W. Health and Hygiene in the Encyclopédie: a medical doctrine for the bourgeoisie. *J Hist Med* 1974; **29**: 399-421; Laignel-Lavastine M. Les médecins collaborateurs de l'Encyclopédie. *Revue Hist Sci* 1951; **4**: 353-8; Schwab RN & Rex WE. Inventory of Diderot's Encyclopédie. *Studies on Voltaire and the Eighteenth Century* 1972; **93**: 21-2.

12 *Code Napoléon. Edition Originale et seule officielle.* Paris: de l'Imprimerie Impériale, 1808.

13 Walker N. *Crime and Insanity in England, Volume 1: Historical Perspectives.* Edinburgh: Edinburgh University Press, 1968.

14 Rath G. Neural pathology. A pathogenetic concept of the 18th and 19th Centuries. *Bull Hist Med* 1959; **33**: 526-30. For a wider discussion of Cullen's ideological background see: López Piñero JM. *Historical origins of the concept of neurosis*, translated by D Berrios. Cambridge: Cambridge University Press, 1983; Bowman IA. *William Cullen (1710-90) and the primacy of the nervous system*, Indiana University Ph.D. Thesis, History of Science, Xerox University Microfilms, Ann Arbor, Michigan, 1975; Cottereau MJ. Historique des Nevroses. *La Revue de*

Medecine 1975; **13**: 903-7; Jackson SW. Force and kindred notions in 18thC neurophysiology and medical psychology. *Bulletin Hist Med* 1970; **44**: 397-410, 539-54.

15 Cullen W. *The Works of William Cullen*. Edinburgh: William Blackwood, Vol 2, 1827.

16 Pinel Ph. *Nosographie Philosophique*. 6th edition. Paris: Brosson, 1818.

17 Cohen GD. Historical Views and Evolution of Concepts. In: Reisberg B (ed). *Alzheimer's Disease*. New York: The Free Press, 1963: pp 29-34.

18 Mahendra B. *Dementia*. Lancaster: MTP Press, 1984.

19 Meynert T. Amentia. In: *Klinische Vorlesungen über Psychiatrie auf Wissenschaftlichen Grundlagen, für Studierende und Ärzte, Juristen und Psychologen*. Vienna: Braumüller, 1890. For the history of the term see: Anonymous. Amentia. In: Gräfe CF (ed). *Encyclopädisches Wörterbuch der medicinischen Wissenschaften* Vol 2. JW Boike, Berlin: 1828: 196-206; Pappenheim E. On Meynert's Amentia. *Int J Neurol* 1975; **9**: 310-26.

20 Tomlinson BE & Corsellis JAN. Ageing and the dementias. In: Corsellis JAN, Duchen LW (eds). *Greenfield's Neuropathology* 4th Edition. London: Arnold, 1984: pp 951-1025.

21 Esquirol E. *Des passions*. Paris: Didot Jeune, 1805.

22 Esquirol E. Démence. In: *Dictionaire des Sciences Médicales, par une Société de Médicins et de Chirurgiens*. Paris: Panckouke, 1814: pp 280-93.

23 Bayle LJ. *Traité des Maladies du Cerveau*. Paris: Gabon et Compagnie, 1826.

24 Esquirol E. *Des Maladies Mentales*. Paris: Baillière, 1838.

25 Georget M. *De la Folie*. Paris: Crevot, 1820.

26 Berrios GE. Stupor: a conceptual history. *Psychol Med* 1981; **11**: 677-88. See also: Postel J. Introduction. In: Georget E. *De la Folie*. Paris: Privat, 1972: pp 7-21.

27 Calmeil LF. Démence. In: *Dictionnaire de Médecine on Repertoire General des Sciences Médicales*. 2nd Edition. Paris: Bechet, 1835: pp 70-85.

28 Guislain J. *Traité sur l'aliénation mentale*. Amsterdam: J van der Hey et Fils, 1826.

29 Guislain J. *Leçons orales sur les phrénopathies*. Gand: L. Hebbelynck, 1852.

30 Marc CCH. *De la folie considérée dans ses rapports avec les questions médico-judiciaires*. Paris: Baillière. 2 vols.

31 Morel BA. *Traité des Maladies Mentales*. Paris: Masson, 1860.

32 Crichton A. *An inquiry into the nature and origin of mental derangement. . . 2 Vols*. London: Cadell & Davies, 1798.

33 Coleridge ST. *The philosophical lectures*. Coburn K (ed). London: Pilot Press, 1949.

34 Cauwenbergh LS. J. C. A. Heinroth (1773-1843) A Psychiatrist of the German Romantic Era. *History of Psychiatry*, 1992 (in press).

35 Heinroth JC. *Textbook of Disturbances of Mental life*. Translated by J Schmorak, Vol 2. Baltimore: The Johns Hopkins Press, 1975.

36 Hoffbauer JC. *Médicine légale relative aux aliénés et aux sourds-muets*. Paris: Baillière, 1827.

37 Feuchtersleben Ernst von. *Lehrburch ärztlichen Seelenkunde*. Wien: Carl Gerold, 1845.

38 Feuchtersleben Ernst von. *The Principles of Medical Psychology*. Translated by Lloyd HE, Babington BG. London: Sydenham Society, 1847.

39 Berrios GE. Memory and the cognitive paradigm of dementia during the 19th century: a conceptual history. In Murray RN, Turner TH (eds). *Lectures on the History of Psychiatry*. London: Gaskell, 1990: pp 194-211.

40 Griesinger W. *Die Pathologie und Therapie der psychischen Krankheiten*. 2nd Edition. Stuttgart: Adolf Krabbe, 1861.

41 Krafft-Ebing Rv. De la démence senile. In: *Ann Médico-Psychol* 1876; **34**: 306-7.

42 Krafft-Ebing Rv. *Lehrbuch der Psychiatrie*. 3rd Edition. Stuttgart: Enke, 1888.

43 Kraepelin E. *Lectures on Clinical Psychiatry*. Translated and edited by Thomas Johnstone. London: Tindall and Cox, 1904.

44 Kraepelin E. *Lectures on Clinical Psychiatry*. Revised and edited by Thomas Johnstone, 2nd Edition. London: Baillière, Tindall and Cox, 1906.

45 Kraepelin E. *Psychiatrie: Ein Lehrbuch für Studierende und Ärzte*. Leipzig: Johann Ambrosius Barth, 1910.

46 Ziehen T. Les Démences. In: Marie A (ed). *Traité International de Psychologie Pathologique*. Paris: Alcan, 1911: pp 281-381.

47 Jaspers K. Die Methoden der Intelligenzprüfung und der Begriff der Demenz. In: *Zeitschrift für die ges. Neurologie & Psychiatrie* 1910; **1**: 402-52.

48 Jaspers K. *Allgemeine Psychopathologie*, 5th Edition. Berlin: Springer, 1948.

49 Salmon W. *Iatrica: Seu Praxis Medendi*, 3rd Edition. London: Rolls, 1694.

50 D'Assigny M. *The Art of Memory*. London: Bell, 1706.

51 Prichard JC. *A Treatise on Insanity and other Disorders Affecting the Mind*. London: Sherwood, Gilbert and Piper, 1835.

52 Bucknill JC, Tuke DH. *A Manual of Psychological Medicine*. London: Churchill, 1858.

53 Berrios GE. Negative and positive signals: A conceptual history. In: Marneros A *et al* (eds). *Negative versus Positive Schizophrenia*. Berlin: Springer, 1991 (in press).

54 Taylor J (ed). *Selected Writings of John Hughlings Jackson*. 2 vols. London: Hodder and Stoughton, 1931.

55 Constantinidis J, Richard J, Ajuariaguerra J de. Dementias with senile plaques and neurofibrillary changes. In: Isaacs AD, Post F (eds). *Studies in Geriatric Psychiatry*. Chichester: Wiley & Sons, 1978, pp 119-52.

56 Maudsley H. *The Pathology of Mind*. London: MacMillan and Co, 1895.

57 Clouston TS. *Clinical Lectures on Mental Diseases*, 2nd Edition. London: Churchill, 1887.

58 Todd J, Ashworth AL. The West Riding Asylum and James Crichton-Browne, 1818-76. In: Berrios GE, Freeman H (eds). *150 Years of British Psychiatry, 1841-1991*. London: Gaskell, 1991: pp 389-418.

59 Browne JC. Clinical lectures on mental and cerebral diseases. *BMJ* 1874; **i**: 601-5.

60 Savage GH. *Insanity and Allied Neuroses: Practical and Clinical*, 2nd Edition. London: Cassell & Company, 1886.

61 *The Nomenclature of Diseases. Drawn up by the Royal College of Physicians*, 4th Edition. London: Darling & Son, 1906.

62 Bolton JS. The histological basis of amentia and dementia. *Arch Neurol* 1903; **2**: 424-612.

63 Hinsie LE, Campbell RJ. *Psychiatric Dictionary*, 4th Edition. New York: Oxford University Press. 1970.

64 Creutzfeldt HG. Über eine eigenartigeherdförmige Erkrankung des Zentralnervensystems. *Zeitschrift ges Neurol Psychiat* 1920; **57**: 1-18.

65 Economo C von. *Encephalitis Lethargica: Its Sequelae and Treatment*. Translated and adapted by Newman KO. London: Oxford University Press, 1931.

66 Critchley M. Pre-senile psychoses. *Proc Roy Soc Med* 1938; **31**: 1447-53.

67 Mayer Gross W. Arteriosclerotic, senile and presenile psychoses. In: Fleming GWTH (ed). *Recent Progress in Psychiatry*, Vol 1, Journal of Mental Science. London: Churchill, 1944: pp 316-27.

68 Maulitz RC. *Morbid appearances. The anatomy of pathology in the early nineteenth century*. Cambridge: Cambridge University Press, 1987.

69 Berrios GE. The psychopathology of affectivity: conceptual and historical aspects. *Psychol Med* 1985; **15**: 745-58.

70 Berrios GE. The psychiatry of old age: a conceptual history. In: Copeland JRM *et al* (eds). *The Psychiatry of Old Age*. New York: Wiley, 1992 (in press).

71 Ackerknecht EH. *Medicine at the Paris Hospital 1794-1848*. Baltimore: Johns Hopkins Press, 1967.

72 Pick D. *Faces of Degeneration. A European disorder 1848-1918*. Cambridge: Cambridge University Press, 1989.

73 Kevles D. *In the Name of Eugenics: Genetics and the Uses of Human Heredity*. New York: Wiley, 1985. For wider aspects

see: Morton P. *The Vital Sciences: Biology and the Literary Imagination 1860-1900*. London: Allen & Unwin, 1984.

74 Berrios GE. see 39.

Chapter 3
Alzheimer and His Time

1   Amaducci LA, Rocca WA, Schoenberg BS. Origin of the distinction between Alzheimer's disease and senile dementia: how history can clarify nosology. *Neurology* 1986; **36**: 1497-9.

2   Beach Th. The history of Alzheimer's Disease: three debates. *J Hist Med Allied Sci* 1987; **42**: 327-49.

3   Bick K, Amaducci L (eds). *Alzheimer's First Case Rediscovered*. Padova: Liviana Press, 1989.

4   Cohen GD. Historical views and evolution of concepts. In: Reisberg B (ed). *Alzheimer's Disease*. New York: The Free Press, 1983: pp 29-43.

5   Hoff P, Hippius H. Alois Alzheimer. Ein überblick über Leben und Werk anlässlich seines 125. Geburtstages. *Nervenarzt* 1989; **60**: 332-7.

6   Kreutzberg GW, Gudden W. Alois Alzheimer. *Trends Neurosci* 1988; **11**: 256-7.

7   Meyer JE. Alois Alzheimer. In: Kolle K (ed). *Grosse Nervenärzte*. Vol 2. Stuttgart: Thieme, 1959: pp 32-8.

8   Lewey FH. Alois Alzheimer. In: Haymaker W, Schiller F (eds). *The Founders of Neurology*. Springfield, Ill: Thomas, 1953: pp 315-9.

9   Robinson RA. The evolution of geriatric psychiatry. *Med Hist* 1972; **16**: 184-93.

10 Thomas M, Isaac M. Alois Alzheimer. A memoir. *Trends Neurosci* 1987; **10**: 306-7.

11 Zeman FD. Life's later years—studies in the medical history of old age; part XI: The nineteenth century. *J Mt Sinai Hosp* 1947; **13**: 241-56.

12 Zeman FD. Life's later years—studies in the medical history of old age; part XII: The nineteenth century (concluded). *J Mt Sinai Hosp* 1950; **17**: 53-68.

13 Dillman R. *Alzheimer's Disease*. Amsterdam: Thesis, 1990.

14 Ueber die Ohrenschmalzdruesen. *Med Diss* University of Wurzburg, 1888.

15 Alzheimer's leaving-certificate of the Royal Humanistic Gymnasium in Aschaffenburg; July 14, 1883 (unpublished).

16 Kraepelin E. Lebenserinnerungen. Hippius H, Peters G, Ploog D (eds). Berlin, Heidelberg, New York: Springer, 1983. English edition: *Memoirs*. Berlin, Heidelberg, New York: Springer, 1987.

17 Kraepelin E. Lebensschicksale deutscher Forscher (Alzheimer, Brodmann, Nissl). *Mnchn med Wschr* 1920; **67**: 75-8.

18 Histologische Studien zur Differenzialdiagnose der progressiven
    Paralyse. *Histol. u. histopathol. Arbeiten uber die Grosshirnrinde
    mit besonderer Bercksichtigung der path. Anat. der Geistes-
    krankheiten* 1904; **1**: 18-314.
19 Berrios GE. Dementia during the seventeenth and eighteenth
    centuries: a conceptual history. *Psychol Med* 1987; **17**:
    829-37.
20 Janzarik W. Forschungsrichtungen und Lehrmeinungen in der
    Psychiatrie: Geschichte, Gegenwart, forensische Bedeutung. In:
    Göppinger H, Witter H (eds). *Handbuch der forensischen
    Psychiatrie*. Berlin, Heidelberg, New York: Springer, 1972:
    pp 588-662.
21 Die diagnostischen Schwierigkeiten in der Psychiatrie. *Zschr
    ges Neurol Psychiat* 1910; **1**: 1-19.
22 Conolly J. *The Treatment of the Insane Without Mechanical
    Restraints*. London: Smith, Elder & Co, 1856.
23 25 Jahr Psychiatrie. Ein Rückblick anlässlich des 25-jührigen
    Jubilaums von Prof. Dr. Emil Sioli als Direktor der Frankfurter
    Irrenanstalt. *Arch Psychiatr Nervenkrankh* 1913; **52**:
    853-66.
24 Ueber einen Fall von spinaler progressiver Muskelatrophie mit
    hinzutretender Erkrankung bulbärer Kerne und der Rinde.
    Arch Psychiatr Nervenkrankh 1892; **23**: 459-85.
25 Die Paralysis progressiva der Entwicklungsjahre. *Neurol Zbl*
    1894; **13**: 732.
26 Die arteriosklerotische Atrophie des Gehirns. *Allg Zschr
    Psychiatr u psychisch-gerichtl Med* 1895; **51**: 809-12.
27 Ueber die durch Druck auf den Augapfel hervorgerufenen
    Visionen. *Zbl Nervenheilk Psychiatr* 1895; **18** (Neue Folge 6 Bd.):
    473-8.
28 Die Frühform der allgemeinen progressiven Paralyse. *Allg Zschr
    Psychiatr u psychisch-gerichtl Med* 1896; **52**: 533-94.
29 Ueber die anatomische Ausbreitung des paralytischen De-
    generationsprozesses. *Neurol Zbl* 1896; **15**: 1007.
30 Ein 'geborener Verbrecher'. *Arch Psychiatr Nervenkrankh* 1896;
    28: 327-353.
31 Funf Falle, in welchen sich neben einer hochgradigen Arterio-
    sklerose der Gefässe disseminierte Herde in der Rinde, den
    Markleisten und im tiefen Mark finden. *Zbl Nervenheilk
    Psychiatr* 1896; **19** (Neue Folge 7 Bd.): 549.
32 Beitrag zur patologischen Anatomie der Hirnrinde und zur
    anatomischen Grundlage einiger Psychosen. *Mschr Psychaitr
    Neurol* 1897; **2**: 82-120.
33 Ein Fall von luetischer Meningomyelitis und-Encephalitis. *Arch
    Psychiatr Nervenkrankh* 1897; **29**: 63-79.
34 Ueber perivasculäre Gliose. *Allg Zschr Psychiatr u psychisch-
    geritchtl Med* 1897; **53**: 863-5.

35 Ueber rückschreitende Amnesie bei der Epilepsie. *Zbl Nervenheilk Psychiatr* **20** (Neue Folge 8 Bd.): 316-7 and *Allg Zschr Psychiatr u psychisch-gerichtl Med* 1897; **53**: 483-99.

36 Das Delirium acutum. *Mschr Psychiatr Neurol* 1897; **2**: 64-65 und *Arch Psychiatr Nervenkrankh* 1897; **29**: 1019-20.

37 Die Colloidentartung des Gehirns. *Arch Psychiatr Nervenkrankh* 1898; **30**: 18-53 and *Neurol Cbl* 1895; **14**: 886.

38 Neuere Arbeiten über die Dementia senilis und die auf atheromatöser Gefässerkrankung basierenden Gehirnkrankheiten (1898). *Mschr Psychiatr Neurol* 1898; **3**: 101-15.

39 Ein Beitrag zur patholigischen Anatomie der Epilepsie. *Mschr Psychiatr Neurol* 1898; **4**: 345-69.

40 Beitrag zur pathologischen Anatomie der Geistesstörungen des Greisenalters. *Neurol Zbl* 1899; **18**: 95-6.

41 Einiges zur pathölogischen Anatomie der chronischen Geistesstörungen. *Allg Zschr Psychiatr u psychisch-gerichtl Med* 1900; **57**: 597-9.

42 Ueber atypische Paralysen. *Allg Zschr Psychiatr u psychisch-gerichtl Med* 1902; **59**: 170-4 and *Mschr Psychiatr Neurol* 1902; **11**: 73-5.

43 Die Seelenstörungen auf arteriosklerotischer Grundlage. *Allg Zschr Psychiatr u psychisch-gerichtl Med* 1902; **59**: 695-711.

44 Spielmeyer W. Alzheimers Lebenswerk. *Zschr ges Neurol Psychiat* 1916; **33**: 1-41.

45 Kraepelin E. *Die Abschaffung des Strafmasses*. Stuttgart: Enke, 1888.

46 Lombroso C. *L'uomo delinquente in rapporto alla antropologia, alla giurisprudenza ed alle discipline carceria*. Milano, 1876.

47 Lewis A. "Endogenous" and "exogenous" a useful dichotomy? *Psychol Med* 1971 **1**: 191-6.

48 Gaston A, Tatarelli R. Analyse critique de l'évolution du concept d'endogéne. *L'Evolution Psychiatrique* 1984; **49**: 569-75.

49 Hermle L. Die Degenerationslehre in der Psychiatrie. *Fortschr Neurol Psychiat* 1986; **54**: 69-79.

50 Pick D. *Faces of Degeneration—A European Disorder 1848-1918*. Cambridge: Cambridge University Press, 1989.

51 Genil-Perrin G. *Histoire des origins et de l'évolution de l'idée de dégénérescence in médicine mental*. Paris: Leclerc, 1913.

52 Einiges über die anatomischen Grundlagen der Idiotie. *Zbl Nervenheilk Psychiat* 1904; **27** (Neue Folge 15 Bd.): 497-505.

53 Ueber die Indikation für eine künstliche Schwangerschaftsunterbrechung bei Geisteskranken. *Mnchn med Wschr* 1907; **54**: 1617-21.

54 Die Gruppierung der Epilepsie. *Allg Zschr Psychiatr u psychisch-gerichtl Med* 1907; **64**: 418-21.

55 Zur Frage der Spätepilepsie. *Zschr ges Neurol Psychiat* 1913; (Ref.) **7**: 82-3.

56 Uber den gegenwartigen Stand der Lehre von der Epilepsie. *Dtsch Med Wschr* 1913; **39**: 1451.

57 Ist die Einrichtung einer psychiatrischen Abteilung im Reichsgesundheitsamt erstrebenswert? *Zschr ges Neurol Psychiat* 1911; **6**: 242-6.

58 Kraepelin E. Ein Forschungsinstitut für Psychiatrie. *Zschr ges Neurol Psychiat* 1916; **32**: 1-38.

59 Über einen eigenartigen, schweren Erkrankungsprozess der Hirnrinde. *Neurol Zbl* 1906; **25**: 1134 and: Ueber eine eigenartige Erkrankung der Hirnrinde. *Zbl Nervenheilk Psychiat* 1907; **30** (Neue Folge 18 Bd.): 177-9 and: über eine eigenartige Erkrankung der Hirnrinde. *Allg Zschr Psychiat u psychisch-gerichtl Med* 1907; **64**: 146-8.

60 Perusini G. Über klinisch und histologisch eigenartige psychische Erkrankungen des späteren Lebensalters. *Histol u histopathol Arbeiten ueber die Grosshirnrinde mit besonderer Berucksichtigung der path Anat der Geisteskrankheiten* 1910; **3**: 297- 352.

61 Berrios GE. Alzheimer's disease: A conceptual history. *Int J Geriatr Psychiat* 1990; **5**: 355-65.

62 Uber eigenartige Krankheitsflle des spateren Alters *Zschr ges Neurol Psychiat* 1911; **4**: 356-85; also English translation, On certain peculiar diseases of old age. Translated by Förstl H, Levy R. *Hist Psychiatry* 1991; **2**: 71-101.

63 Torak RM. Adult dementia: History, biopsy, pathology. *Neurosurgery* 1979; **4**: 432-4.

64 Fischer O. Miliare Nekrosen mit drusigen Wucherungen der Neurofibrillen, eine regelmässige Veränderung der Hirnrinde bei seniler Demenz. *Mschr Psychiat Neurol* 1907; **22**: 361-72.

65 Haben wir bei den verschiedenen Geisteskrankheiten mit anatomischem Befund einen histologisch annähernd gleichen Krankheitsprocess vorauszusetzen? *Neurol Zbl* 1905; **24**: 680-2 and Uber den Abbau des Nervengewebes. *Allg Zschr Psychiatr u psychisch-gerichtl Med* 1906; **63**: 568-72.

66 Ergebnisse auf dem Gebiete der pathologischen Histologie der Geistesstorungen I. *Zschr ges Neurol Psychiat* 1912; (Ref.) **5**: 753-80.

67 Beitrage zur pathologischen Anatomie der Dementia praecox. *Zschr ges Neurol Psychiat* 1913; (Ref.) **7**: 621-2.

68 The present status of our knowledge of the pathological histology of the cortex in the psychoses. *Am J Insanity* 1913; **70**: 1175 and *Zschr ges Neurol Psychiat* 1914; (Ref.) **8**: 496.

69 Meynert Th. *Psychiatrie. Klinik der Erkrankungen des Vorderhirns.* Wien: Braumüller, 1884.

70 Bresler J. Alzheimers Untersuchungen zur feineren Histologie der Psychosen. *Psych-neurol Wschr* 1911/12; **48**: 479-81.

71 Hoff P. Zum Krankheitsbegriff bei Emil Kraepelin. *Nervenarzt* 1985; **56**: 510-13.

72 Hoff P. Nosologische Grundpostulate bei Emil Kraepelin—
Versuch einer kritischen Wrdigung des Kraepelinschen
Spätwerkes. *Zschr Klin Psychol Psychopathol Psychother* 1988;
36: 328-36.

73 Kraepelin E. *Die Richtungen der psychiatrischen Forschung.*
Leipzig: Vogel, 1887.

74 Berrios GE, Hauser R. The early development of Kraepelin's ideas
on classification: a conceptual history. *Psychol Med* 1988; **18**:
813-21.

75 (Together with AE Hoche). Die Bedeutung der Symptomenkomplexe in der Psychiatrie, besonders im Hinblick auf das
manisch-depressive Irresein. *Zschr ges Neurol Psychiat* 1912;
(Ref.) **5**: 804-10.

76 Hoche AE. Kritisches zur psychiatrischen Formenlehre. *Allg
Zschr Psychiat u psychisch-gerichtl Med* 1906; **63**: 559-63.

77 Hoche AE. Uber die Melancholiefrage. Leipzig, 1910.

78 Kraepelin E. *Psychiatrie*, 5th Edition. Leipzig: Barth, 1896.

79 Birnbaum K. Der Aufbau der Psychose. Ein Klinischer
Versuch. *Allg Zschr Psychiat psychisch-gerichtl Med* 1919; **75**:
455-502.

80 Kraepelin E. Die Erscheinungsformen des Irreseins. *Zschr ges
Neurol Psychiat* 1920; **62**: 1-29.

81 Hoche AE. Die Bedeutung der Symptomenkomplexe in der
Psychiatrie. *Zschr ges Neurol Psychiat* 1912; **12**: 540-51; or
English version, The meaning of symptom complexes in
psychiatry. Translated by Dening TR, Dening DR. *Hist
Psychiatry* 1991 (in press).

82 Wernicke C. Grundriss der Psychiatrie in klinischen Vorlesungen.
2nd edition. Leipzig, 1906.

83 Berrios GE. Presbyophrenia: the rise and fall of a concept.
Psychol Med 1986; **16**: 267-75.

84 Bonhoeffer K. Die symptomatischen Psychosen im Gefolge von
akuten Infektionen und inneren Erkrankungen. Leipzig, Wien:
Deuticke, 1910.

*The references listed below, in addition to those quoted in the text,
constitute Alzheimer's full bibliography*: it is worth noting that
his marriage to the banker's widow made him financially
independent and he was able to supplement his texts with
numerous illustrations.

Das Delirium alcoholicum febrile Magnan's. *Zbl Nervenheilk
Psychiat* 1904; **27** (Neue Folge 15 Bd.): 437-41.

Progressive Paralyse und endarteriitische Hirnlues. *Zbl Nervenheilk
Psychiat* 1905; **28** (Neue Folge 16 Bd.): 443-5.

Zur pathologischen Anatomie der Paralyse und der paralyseahnlichen
Erkrankungen. *Munchn med Wschr* 1906; **53**: 1643-4.

(Together with R Gaupp) Die stationare Paralyse. *Allg Zschr Psychiatr u psychisch-gerichtl Med* 1907; **64**: 656-77.

Einige Methoden zur Fixierung der zelligen Elemente der Cerebrospinalflussigkeit. *Zbl Nervenheilk Psychiat* 1907; **30** (Neue Folge 18 Bd.): 449-51.

Die syphilitischen Geistesstorungen. *Allg Zschr Psychiatr u psychisch-gerichtl Med* 1909; **66**: 920-4 and *Zbl Nervenheilk Psychiatr* 1909; **32** (Neue Folge 20 Bd.); 676-84.

Uber Degeneration und Regeneration an der peripheren Nervenfaser. *Zschr ges Neurol Psychiat* 1910; (Ref.) **1**: 654-5.

Beitrage zur Kenntnis der pathologischen Neuroglia und ihrer Beziehungen zu den Abbauvorgangen im Nervengewebe. *Histol u histopathol Arbeiten uber die Grosshirnrinde mit besonderer Berucksichtigung der path Anat der Geisteskrankheiten* 1910; **3**: 401-562.

Uber die anatomische Grundlage der Huntingtonschen Chorea und der choreatischen Bewegungen uberhaupt. *Zschr ges Neurol Psychiat* 1911; (Ref.) **3**: 566-7.

(Together with Cv Hösslin) Ein Beitrag zur Klinik und patholigischen Anatomie der Westphal-Strümpellschen Pseudosklerose. *Zschr ges Neurol Psychiat* 1912; **8**: 183-209.

Uber noch nicht genauer bekannte paralyseahnliche Krankheitsbilder. *Zschr ges Neurol Psychiat* 1913 (Ref.) **6**: 1074-5.

Residuäre Halluzinose. *Zschr ges Neurol Psychiat* 1913; (Ref.) **7**: 45-6.

Eigenartige metasyphilitische Erkrankung. *Zschr ges Neurol Psychiat* 1913; (Ref.) **7**: 83.

Eigenartiger Verblödungszustand auf arteriosklerotischer Grundlage. *Zschr ges Neurol Psychiat* 1913; (Ref.) **7**: 84-5.

Uber die Abbauvorgänge im Nervensystem. *Zschr ges Neurol Psychiat* 1914; (Ref.) **8**: 81-2.

Uber zwei verschiedene Typen von Entwicklungshemmungen des Gehirns. *Zschr ges Neurol Psychiat* 1914; (Ref.) **8**: 289-90.

Uber einen Fall von Poliomyelitis bulbi et cerebelli. *Zschr ges Neurol Psychiat* 1914; (Ref.) **8**: 534.

Uber einen Fall von "hysterischer Bulbärparalyse". *Zschr ges Neurol Psychiat* 1914; (Ref.) **8**: 534-5.

Fälle von Methylalkoholvergiftung. *Dtsch Med Wschr* 1915; **41**: 635.

Der Krieg und die Nerven. Breslau: Preuss und Jünger, 1915.

Chapter 4
Social Aspects of Alzheimer's Disease

1　Fox P. From senility to Alzheimer's Disease: the rise of the Alzheimer's Disease movement. *Millbank Quarterly* 1989; **67**: 58-102.

2　Townsend P. *The Last Refuge.* London: Routledge & Kegan Paul, 1964.

3   Lewis A. Social causes of admissions to a mental hospital for the aged. *Sociol Rev* 1943; **35**: 86-98.

4   Jimenez MA. *Changing Faces of Madness*. Hanover, NH: University Press of New England, 1987: pp 135, 188.

5   Grob GN. *The State & the Mentally Ill*. Chapel Hill: University of North Carolina Press, 1966: p 346.

6   Notes & News. *J Mental Sci* 1901; **47**: 620-23.

7   Burns BJ, Larson DB, Goldstrom ID, *et al*. Mental disorder among nursing home patients: preliminary findings from the national nursing home survey protest. *Int J Geriatric Psychiatry* 1988; **3**: 27-35.

8   Robertson GM. The prevention of insanity. *J Mental Sci* 1926; **72**: 480-5.

9   Jones K. *A History of the Mental Health Services*. London: Routledge & Kegan Paul, 1972: p 262.

10 Lewis A. Ageing and senility: a major problem in psychiatry. *J Mental Sci* 1946; **92**: 150-70.

11 Anderson F. An historical overview of geriatric medicine: definition and aims. In: Pathy J (ed). *Principles & Practice of Geriatric Medicine*. Chichester: Wiley, 1985.

12 DHSS. Services for Mental Illness Related to Old Age. Circular HM(72)71. London: DHSS 1972.

13 Jolley S, Jolley D. Psychiatric disorders in old age. In: Bennett DH, Freeman HL (eds). *Community Psychiatry: the Principles*. London: Churchill Livingstone, 1991.

14 Kay AWK, Beamish P, Roth M. Old age mental disorders in Newcastle-upon-Tyne: I. Prevalence. *Br J Psychiatry* 1964; **110**: 146-58.

15 O'Connor DW, Pollitt PA, Hyde JB *et al*. The prevalence of dementia as measured by the Cambridge Mental Disorders of the Elderly Examination. *Acta Psych Scand* 1989; **79**: 190-8.

16 Roth M. The principles of providing a service for psychogeriatric patients. In: Wing JK, Hafner H (eds). *Roots of Evaluation*. London: Oxford University Press, 1973.

17 Cooper B. The epidemiological contribution to research on late-life dementia. In: Williams P, Wilkinson G, Raunsley K (eds). *The Scope of Epidemiological Psychiatry*. London: Routledge, 1989: pp 264-86.

18 WHO. *Psychogeriatric Care in the Community*. Public Health in Europe, No. 10. Copenhagen: WHO. London: Croom Helm, 1979.

19 Gurland B, Copeland J, Kuriansky J, Kelleher M, Sharpe L, Dean LL. *The Mind & Mood of Aging*. New York: Haworth Press 1983.

20 Opit LJ. Domiciliary care for the elderly sick: economy or neglect. *BMJ* 1977; **i**: 30-3.

21 O'Connor DW, Pollitt PA, Brook CPB, Reiss BB, Roth M. Does early intervention reduce the number of elderly people with dementia admitted to institutions for long term? *BMJ* 1991; **302**: 871-5.

22 Katzman R, Karasu T. Differential diagnosis of dementia. In: Fields W (ed). *Neurological & Sensory Disorders in the Elderly.* New York: Stratton Intercontinental, 1975: pp 103-4.

23 Gneichen B. Measuring the rising tide. How many dementia cases will there be by 2001? *Br J Psychiatry* 1987; **150**: 193-200.

24 Jorm AF, Kotten AE, Henderson AS. The prevalence of dementia: a quantitative investigation of the literature. *Acta Psych Scand* 1987; **76**: 465-79.

25 Mortimer JA, Schurron LM (eds). *The Epidemiology of Dementia.* New York: Oxford University Press, 1981.

26 Treves T, Kotczyn A, Zilber N *et al.* Presenile dementia in Israel. *Arch Neurol* 1986; **43**: 26-9.

27 Shibayama H, Kasahara Y, Kobayashi H *et al.* Prevalence of dementia in a Japanese elderly population. *Acta Psych Scand* 1986; **74**: 144-51.

28 Shen LG, Chen CH, Zhau YQ, Li SR, Lu M. A three-year follow-up of age-related dementia in an urban area of Beijing. *Acta Psych Scand* 1991; **83**: 99-104.

29 Zheng M, Katzman R, Salmon D *et al.* The prevalence of dementia and Alzheimer's disease in Shanghai, China: impact of age, gender, and education. *Ann Neurol* 1990; **27**: 428-37.

30 Chen DY. Epidemiological survey of stroke in a 700,000 population of Beijing in 1984. Neuroepidemiology Research Workshop, Beijing, 1986. (quoted by Shen *et al*, 1991.)

31 Hagnell O, Lanke J, Rorsman B, Ojesjo L. Does the incidence of age psychosis decrease? *Neuropsychobiology* 1981; **7**: 201-11.

32 Preston GAN. Dementia in elderly adults: prevalence and institutionalisation. *J Gerontology* 1986; **41**: 261-7.

33 Sluss TK, Gruenberg EM, Kramer M. The use of longitudinal studies in the investigation of risk factors for senile dementia-Alzheimer type. In: Mortimer JA, Schurron LM (eds). *The Epidemiology of Dementia.* New York: Oxford University Press, 1981: pp 132-54.

34 Larsson T, Sjogren T, Jacobson G. Senile dementia: a clinical, socio-medical and genetic study. *Acta Psych Scand* 1963; **167** (suppl): 1-259.

35 Heston LL, Mastri AR, Anderson E, White J. Dementia of the Alzheimer type: clinical genetics, natural history and associated conditions. *Arch Gen Psychiatry* 1981; **38**: 1085-90.

36 Mohs RC, Breitner JCS, Silverman JM, Davis KL. Alzheimer's disease: morbid risk among first degree relatives. *Arch Gen Psychiatry* 1987; **44**: 405-8.

37 Breitner JCS. Estimation of familial risk of Alzheimer's disease. *Ann Neurol* 1990; **27**: 338-40.

38 Roth M. Some strategies for tackling the problems of senile demential and related disorders within the next decade. WHO Working Paper IPR/ADR 117 (01)6, 1982.

39 Tomlinson BE, Blessed G, Roth M. Observations on the brains of demented old people. *J Neurol Sci* 1970; **11**: 205-42.

40 Busfield J. *Managing Madness*. London: Hutchinson, 1986: p 369.

41 Caplan G. *Principles of Preventive Psychiatry*. London: Tavistock, 1964.

42 Bennett DH, Freeman HL. Principles and prospect. In: Bennett DH, Freeman HL (eds). *Community Psychiatry: the Principles*. London: Churchill Livingstone, 1991: pp 3-4.

Chapter 5
The Vascular Dementias

1 Meyer JS *et al* (eds). *Vascular and Multi-Infarct Dementia*. New York: Futura Publishing, 1988.

2 Hachinski VC, Lassen NA, Marshall J. Multi-infarct dementia. A cause of mental deterioration in the elderly. *Lancet* 1974; **ii**: 207-10.

3 Duret H. Recherches anatomiques sur la circulation de l'encephale. *Arch Physiol* (Paris), 2nd Series 1874; **1**: 60-91; 316-53; 664-93; 919-57.

4 Wright-St Clair RE. *Doctors Monro: A Medical Saga*. London: The Wellcome Historical Medical Library, 1964.

5 Comrie JD. *History of the Scottish Medicine to 1860*. London: Baillière, Tindall & Cox, 1927.

6 Hill L. *The Physiology and Pathology of the Cerebral Circulation*. London: J & A Churchill, 1896. For a review of views on circulatory physiology in the insane before Hill see: Greenless TD. A contribution to the study of diseases of the circulatory system in the insane. *J Ment Sci* 1885; **31**: 327-55.

7 Thompson J (ed). *The Works of William Cullen*. Vol 1. Edinburgh: Blackwood, 1827: p 293; See also Chapter 2, ref. 14.

8 Cullen, *vide* 7, Vol 2, p 164.

9 Bayle ALJ. *Traité des Maladies du Cerveau*. Paris: Gabon, 1826.

10 Rostan L. *Recherches sur le Ramollissement du Cerveau*. 2nd Edition. Paris: Bechet, 1823. On history of stroke see: Schiller F. Concepts of stroke before and after Virchow. *Medical Hist* 1970; **14**: 115-31 and Fields WF, Lermak NA. *A History of Stroke*. New York: Oxford University Press, Chapter 1.

11 Rostan, *vide* 9.

12 Durand-Fardel M. *Traité du Ramollissement du Cerveau*. Paris: Baillière, 1843.

13 Grmek MD. On ageing and old age. In: Bodenheimer FS, Weisbach WW (eds). *Monographie Biologicae*. Den Haag: Uitgerverij Dr W Junk, 1958. For a specific cellular theory see: Marinesco G. Mécanisme de la sénilité et de la mort des cellules nerveuses. *Comptes Rendus Hebdomadaires des Seances de L'Academie des Sciences* 1900; **130**: 1136-9.

14 Long ER. The development of our knowledge of arteriosclerosis. In: Cawdry EV (ed). *Arteriosclerosis*. New York: MacMillan, 1933: pp 19-52.

15 Walton GL. Arteriosclerosis probably not an important factor in the etiology and prognosis of involution psychoses. *Boston Med Surg J* 1912; **167**: 834-6.

16 Mayer-Gross W. Arteriosclerotic, senile and presenile psychoses. *J Ment Sci* 1944; **1**: 316-27.

17 Rostan, *vide* 9.

18 Durand-Fardel, *vide* 12.

19 Jackson JH. A lecture on softening of the brain. *Lancet* 1875; **ii**: 335-9.

20 For an account of the concept of dissolution see: Dewhurst K. *Hughlings Jackson on Psychiatry*. Oxford: Sandford Publications, 1982, and López Piñero JM. *John Hughlings Jackson (1835-1911)*. Madrid: Moneda, 1973.

21 Ball B, Chambard E. Démence. In: Dechambre A, Lereboullet L (eds). *Dictionnaire Encyclopédique des Sciences Médicales*. Paris: Masson, 1881: pp 559-605.

22 Charcot JM. *Clinical Lectures on Senile and Chronic Diseases*. London: The New Sydenham Society, 1881.

23 Barret AM. Pre-senile arteriosclerotic and senile disorders of the brain and cord. In: White WA, Jellife SE (eds). *The Modern Treatment of Nervous and Mental Diseases*. London: Henry Kimpton, 1913: pp xx.

24 Marie A. *La Démence*. Paris: Doin, 1906.

25 Southard EE. Anatomical findings in senile dementia: A diagnostic study bearing especially on the group of cerebral atrophies. *Am J Insanity* 1910; **61**: 673-708.

26 Olah G. Was kann man heute unter Arteriosklerotischen Psychosen verstehen? *Psych Neur Wochenschr* 1910; **52**: 532-3.

27 Binswanger O *et al* (eds). *Lehrbuch der Psychiatre*. Jena: Gustav Fischer, 1915.

28 North HM, Bostock F. Arteriosclerosis and mental disease. *J Ment Sci* 1925; **71**: 600-1. See also: Phillips JGP. Psychoses associated with senility and arterio-sclerosis. In: *Early Mental Disease. The Lancet* Extra Numbers Nº 2. London: Wakley & Son, 1912: pp 146-8.

29 Claude H. *Précis de Pathologie Interne. Maladies du Système Nerveux (1)*. Paris: Baillière, 1922.

30 Claude H, Cuel F. Cerebral starvation due to premature arterio-sclerosis, without focal ischaemia. *J Ment Sci* 1927; **73**: 676-7.

31 Vallejo Nágera A. *Tratado de Psiquiatría*. Barcelona: Salvat, 1954. The same views are found in French (e.g. Ey H *et al*. *Manuel de Psychiatrie*. Paris: Masson, 4th Edition, 1974), German (e.g. Benda ClE *et al*. *Klinische Psychiatrie*, Berlin: Springer, 1960), and British textbooks (e.g. Slater E, Roth M. *Clinical Psychiatry*. 3rd Edition, London: Baillière, 1969).

32 Mental Disorders: *Glossary and Guide to their Classification in accordance with the Ninth Revision of the International Classification of Diseases*. Geneva: World Health Organisation, 1978.

33 Hounsfield GN. Computerised transverse axial scanning (tomography): Part 1. Description of system. *Br J Radiol* 1973; **46**: 1016-22.

34 Marshall J. Vascular and multi-infarct dementia. Do they exist? In: Meyer JS *et al* (eds). *Vascular and Multi-Infarct Dementia*. New York: Futura Publishing, 1988: pp 1-4.

35 Tomlinson BE, Corsellis JAN. Ageing and the dementias. In: Adams JH *et al* (eds). *Greenfield's Neuropathology*. London: Arnold, 1984, pp 951-1025.

36 Neary D *et al*. Single photon emission tomography using 99mTc-HM-PAO in the investigation of dementia. *J Neurol Neurosurg Psychiatry* 1987; **50**: 1101-9.

37 see chapter on 'History of Subcortical Dementia' (this book).

38 Kristensen MO. Progressive supranuclear palsy—20 years later. *Acta Neurol Scand* 1985; **71**: 177-89.

Chapter 6
The History of Subcortical Dementia

1 Berrios GE. Dementia during the 17th and 18th centuries: a conceptual history. *Psychol Med* 1987; **17**: 829-37.

2 Berrios GE. Memory and the cognitive paradigm of dementia during the 19th century. In: Murray RN, Turner TH (eds). *Lectures on the History of Psychiatry*. London: Gaskell, 1990: 194-211.

3 Berrios GE. Alzheimer's disease: a conceptual history. *Int J Geriat Psychiat* 1990; **5**: 355-65.

4 Von Stockert FG. Subcorticale Demenz. *Arch Psychiat* 1932; **97**: 77-100.

5 Mandell AM, Albert ML. History of subcortical dementia. In: Cummings JL (ed). *History of Subcortical Dementia*. New York: Oxford University Press, 1990: 17-30.

6 Mayeux R, Stern Y, Rosen J, Benson DF. Is "subcortical dementia" a recognizable clinical entity? *Ann Neurol* 1983; **14**: 278-80.

7 Mental Disorders: *Glossary and Guide to their classification in accordance with the ninth revision of the international classification of diseases.* Geneva: World Health Organisation, 1978.

8 American Psychiatric Association: *Diagnostic and Statistical Manual of Mental Disorders*, 3rd Edition, revised. Washington DC: American Psychiatric Association, 1978.

9 Cummings JL, Benson DF. Subcortical dementia—review of an emerging concept. *Arch Neurol* 1984; **41**: 874-9.

10 Whitehouse PJ. The concept of subcortical and cortical dementia: another look. *Neurol Progress* 1986; **19**: 1-6.

11 Cummings JL, Benson DF. Subcortical dementias in the extrapyramidal disorders. Chapter 4 in: *Dementia—a clinical approach.* Boston: Butterworths, 1983: pp 73-124.

12 Bleuler E. *Textbook of Psychiatry.* Brill AA (trans.) New York: MacMillan Co, 1924.

13 Bleuler M. Psychiatry of cerebral disease. *BMJ* 1951; **2**: 1233-8.

14 Naville F. Études sur les complications et les sequelles mentales de l'encephalite epidemique—la bradyphrenie. *L'Encéphale* 1922; **17**: 369-75; 433-6.

15 Parkinson J. *An Essay on the Shaking Palsy.* London: Sherwood, Neely and Jones, 1817.

16 Yahr MD. A physician for all seasons—James Parkinson 1755-1824. *Arch Neurol* 1978; **35**: 185-8.

17 Jefferson M. James Parkinson 1755-1824. *BMJ* 1973; **2**: 601-3.

18 Parkinson G. *Madhouses: Observations of the Act Regulating Mad-houses.* London: Whittingham, 1811.

19 McMenemey WH. A note on James Parkinson as a reformer of the lunacy acts. *Proc Roy Soc Med* 1955; **48**: 593-4.

20 Huntington G. On chorea. *Med Surg Reporter* 1872; **26**: 317-21.

21 Hayden MR. *Huntington's Chorea.* Berlin: Springer Verlag, 1981.

22 Elliotson J. St Vitus's dance. *Lancet* 1832; **i**: 162-5.

23 Dunglison R. *The Practice of Medicine*, 1st Edition. Philadelphia: Lee and Blanchard, 1842.

24 Dunglison R. *The Practice of Medicine*, 3rd Edition. Philadelphia: Lee and Blanchard, 1848.

25 Lyon IW. Chronic hereditary chorea. *Am Med Times* 1863; **7**: 289-90.

26 Wood GB. *A Treatise on the Practice of Medicine.* Philadelphia: Lippincott, Grambo, 1855.

27 De Jong RN. George Huntington and his relationship to the earlier descriptions of chronic hereditary chorea. *Ann Med History* 1937; **9**: 201-10.

28 Huber A. Chorea hereditaria der Erwachsenen (Huntington'sche Chorea). *Virchows Arch Pathol Anat* 1887; **108**: 267-85.

29 Bruyn GW, Baro F, Myrianthopoulos NC. *Centennial Bibliography of Huntington's Chorea 1872-1972.* Louvain: Leuven University Press and Martinus Nijhoff, 1974.

30 Binswanger O. Die Abgrenzung der allgemeinen progressiven Paralyse. *Berliner Klin Wochenschr* 1894; **32**: 1180-6.

31 Olszewski J. Subcortical arteriosclerotic encephalopathy: review of the literature on the so-called Binswanger's disease and presentation of two cases. *World Neur* 1962; **3**: 357-75.

32 Alzheimer A. Die Seelenstörungen auf arteriosclerotischer Grundlage. *Ztschr Psychiat (Berlin)* 1902; **59**: 695-711.

33 Berger H. Otto Binswanger (obituary) *Arch Psychiat Nervenkr* 1929; **89**: 1-10.

34 De Reuck J, Schaumburg HH. Periventricular atherosclerotic leuko-encephalopathy. *Neurol* 1972; **22**: 1094-7.

35 Lotz PR, Ballinger WE, Quisling RG. Subcortical arteriosclerotic encephalopathy: CT spectrum and pathological correlation. *Am J Radiol* 1986; **147**: 1209-14.

36 Hachinski VC, Potter P, Merskey H. Leuco-araiosis. *Arch Neurol* 1987; **44**: 21-3.

37 Drayer BP. Imaging of the aging brain. *Radiology* 1988; **166**: 785-806.

38 Hachinski VC, Lassen NA, Marshall J. Multi-infarct dementia—a cause of mental deterioration in the elderly. *Lancet* 1974; **2**: 207-10.

39 Wilson SAK. Progressive lenticular degeneration: a familial nervous disease associated with cirrhosis of the liver. *Brain* 1912; **34**: 295-509.

40 Birch CA. Kinnier Wilson's disease and Wilson's sign. *Practitioner* 1974; **212**: 263-4.

41 Pfeifer B. Psychic disturbance occurring in brain tumours. *Arch Psychiat Nervenkr* 1910; **47**: 558.

41 Smyth GE, Stern K. Tumours of the thalamus—a clinico-pathological study. *Brain* 1938; **61**: 339-74.

42 *Proceedings of the Royal Society of Medicine*. London: 1931; **24**: 997-1008.

43 Hallervorden J, Spatz H. Eigenartige Erkrankung im extra-pyramidalen System mit besonderer Beteiligung des Globus pallidus und der Substantia nigra. *Ztschr Ges Neurol* 1922; **79**: 254.

44 Bebb GL. A study of memory deterioration in encephalitis lethargica. *J Nerv Ment Dis* 1925; **61**: 356-65.

45 Kasanin J, Crank RP. A case of extensive calcification of the brain. *Arch Neurol Psychiat* 1935; **34**: 164-78.

46 Stern K. Severe dementia associated with bilateral symmetrical degeneration of the thalamus. *Brain* 1939; **62**: 157-71.

47 Grunthal E. Über thalamische Demenz. *Monatsschr Psychiat Neurol* 1942; **106**: 114-28.

48 Davison C, Brill NQ. Essential hypertension and chronic hypertensive encephalopathy. *Ann Intern Med* 1939; **12**: 1766-81.

49 Hirano A, Kurland LT *et al.* Parkinsonism-dementia complex. An endemic disease on the Island of Guam. *Brain* 1961; **84**: 642-79.
50 Greenfield JG. *The Spino-Cerebellar Degenerations.* Oxford: Blackwell Scientific Publications, 1954.
51 Cummings JL, Benson DF. Dementia in vascular and infectious disorders. Chapter 5 in: Cummings JL & Benson DF (eds). *Dementia—A Clinical Approach.* Boston: Butterworths, 1983: pp 125-67.
52 Richardson JC, Steele JC, Olszewski J. Supranuclear ophthalmoplegia, pseudobulbar palsy, nuchal dystonia and dementia. *Trans Am Neurol Assoc* 1963; **88**: 25-7.
53 Posey WC. Paralysis of the upward movements of the eye. *Ann Ophthal* 1904; **13**: 523-9.
54 Steele JC. Progressive supranuclear palsy. *Brain* 1972; **95**: 693-704.
55 Albert ML, Feldman RG, Willis AL. The subcortical dementia of progressive supranuclear palsy. *J Neurol Neurosurg Psychiat* 1974; **37**: 121-30.
56 Neumann MA, Cohn R. Progressive subcortical gliosis, a rare form of presenile dementia. *Brain* 1967; **90**: 405-17.

Chapter 7
Other Forms of Dementia

1 Bayle ALJ. *Recherches sur les maladies mentales.* Paris: Thèse de Médecine, 1822.
2 Hare E. The origin and spread of dementia paralytica. *J Ment Sci* 1959; **105**: 594-626.
3 Zilboorg G. *A history of medical psychology.* New York: Norton & Company, 1941.
4 Dörner K. *Bürger und Irre.* Frankfurt: Verlagsanstalt, 1969.
5 Ackernknecht E. *Kürze Geschichte der Psychiatrie.* Stuttgart: Enke, 1957.
6 Berrios GE. 'Depressive pseudodementia' or 'melancholic dementia': a 19th century view. *J Neurol Neurosurg Psychiatry* 1985; **48**: 393-400.
7 Bercheri P. *Les Fondements de la Clinique.* Paris: La Bibliothèque d'Ornicar, 1980.
8 Baillarger J. Sur la Théorie de la Paralysie Générale. *Ann Médico-Psychol* 1883; **41**: 18-52; 191-218.
9 Fournier A. *Syphilis du Cerveau.* Paris: Baillière, 1875.
10 Baillarger J. Doit-on dans la classification des maladies mentales assigner une place à part aux pseudo-paralysies générales? *Ann Médico-Psychol* 1883; **41**: 521-5.
11 Postel J. 'La paralysie générale. In: Postel J, Quétel C (eds). *Nouvelle Histoire de la Psychiatrie.* Toulouse: Privat, 1983.
12 Report Association of German physicians practising in lunacy. *BMJ* 1883; **ii**: 1198-9.

13 Morel BA. *Études Cliniques sur les Maladies Mentales.* 2 Vols. Paris: Masson, 1852.

14 Kraepelin E. *Dementia Praecox and Paraphrenia*, translation by R. M. Barclay. Edinburgh: Livingstone, 1919.

15 Bleuler E. *Dementia praecox oder Gruppe der Schizophrenien.* Leipzig: Franz Deuticke, 1911.

16 Schneider K. *Clinical Psychopathology*, translation by M. W. Hamilton. New York: Grune & Stratton, 1959.

17 Hoenig J. The concept of schizophrenia: Kraepelin-Bleuler-Schneider. *Br J Psychiatry* 1983; **142**: 547-56.

18 Rieder RO. The origins of our confusion about schizophrenia. *Psychiatry* 1974; **37**: 197-208.

19 Berrios GE. Introduction to 1911: Eugen Bleuler. In: Thompson C (ed). *The Origins of Modern Psychiatry.* New York: Wiley, 1987: pp 200-209.

20 Ellard J. Did schizophrenia exist before the eighteenth century. *Aust NZ J Psychiatry* 1987; **21**: 306-14.

21 Jeste DV, del Carmen R, Lohr JB, Wyatt RJ. Did schizophrenia exist before the eighteenth century. *Compr Psychiatry* 1985; **26**: 493-503.

22 Klaf FS, Hamilton JG. Schizophrenia—a hundred years ago and today. *J Ment Sci* 1961; **128**: 819-27.

23 Hare E. Schizophrenia before 1800? The case of the Revd George Trosse. *Psychol Med* 1988; **18**: 279-85.

24 Hare E. Schizophrenia as a different disease. *Br J Psychiatry* 1988; **153**: 521-31.

25 Boyle M. Is schizophrenia what it was? A re-analysis of Kraepelin's and Bleuler's population. *J Hist Behav Sci* 1990; **26**: 323-33.

26 Carpenter PK. Descriptions of schizophrenia in the psychiatry of Georgian Britain: John Haslam and James Tilly Matthews. *Compr Psychiatry* 1989; **30**: 332-8.

27 Wender PH. Dementia praecox: the development of a concept. *Am J Psychiatry* 1963; **119**: 1143-51.

28 Baruk H. *La psychiatrie française de Pinel à nos jours.* Paris: Presses Universitaires de France, 1967.

29 Kahlbaum KL. *Die Katatonie.* Berlin: Kirschwald, 1874.

30 Jung CG. *Über die Psychologie der Dementia praecox: Ein Versuch.* Falle: Carl Marhold, 1907.

31 Lanteri-Laura G, Gros M. *La Discordance.* Paris: Unicet, 1984.

32 Berrios GE, Hauser R. The early development of Kraepelin's ideas on classification: a conceptual history. *Psychol Med* 1988; **18**: 813-21.

33 Berrios GE. History of the functional psychoses. *Br Med Bull* 1987; **43**: 484-98.

34 Johnstone E, Crow TJ, Frith CD *et al.* The dementia of dementia praecox. *Acta Psych Scand* 1978; **57**: 305-24.

35 Kiloh LG. Pseudo-dementia. *Acta Psych Scand* 1961; **37**: 336-51.

36 Wells CE. Pseudodementia. *Am J Psychiatry* 1979; **136**: 895-900.

37 Caine ED. Pseudodementia. *Arch Gen Psychiatry* 1981; **38**: 1359-64.

38 Bulbena A, Berrios GE. Pseudodementia: facts and figures. *Br J Psychiatry* 1986; **148**: 87-94.

39 Mairet A. *De la démence melancolique*. Paris: Masson, 1883.

40 Ganser SJM. Über eine eigenartigen hysterischen Dämmer-zustand. *Arch Psychiatrie Nervenkrankheiten* 1898; **30**: 635-40; 654-5.

41 Nitsche P, Wilmanns K. *The History of Prison Psychoses*. New York: J Nerv Ment Dis Pubs Co, 1912.

42 Ball B, Chambard E. 'Démence'. In: Dechambre A (ed). *Dictionnaire Encyclopédique du Sciences Médicales*. Vol 26. Paris: Asselin, 1882.

43 Cotard J. Du délire des negations. *Arch Neurol* 1882; **4**: 152-170; 282-96.

44 Dumas G. *Les états intellectuels dans la mélancolie*. Paris: Alcan, 1894.

45 Bleuler E. *Textbook of Psychiatry*. New York: MacMillan, 1934.

46 Madden JJ, Luhan JA, Kaplan LA *et al*. Non-dementing psychoses in older persons. *J Am Med Assoc* 1952; **150**: 1567-70.

47 Anderson EW, Tgrethowan WH, Kenna JC. An experimental investigation of simulation and pseudodementia. *Acta Psych Neurol Scand* 1959; **34** (Suppl 132).

48 Kahlbaum KL. *Die Gruppierung der psychischen Krankheiten*. Danzig: AW Kafemann, 1863.

49 Fischer O. Ein weiterer Beitrag zur Klinik und Pathologie der presbyophrenen Demenz. *Zeit gesamte Neurol Psychiatrie* 1912; **12**: 99-135.

50 Lanczik M. *Der Breslauer Psychiater Carl Wernicke*. Sigmaringen: Thorbecke, 1988.

51 Berrios GE. Presbyophrenia: the rise and fall of a concept. *Psychol Med* 1986; **16**: 267-75.

52 Berrios GE. Presbyophrenia: clinical aspects. *Br J Psychiatry* 1985; **147**: 76-9.

53 Rouby J. *Contribution à l'étude de la presbyophrénie*. Thèse de Médicine. Paris: E Nourris, 1911.

54 Truelle V, Bessière R. Recherches sur la presbyophrénie. *L'Encéphale* 1911; **6**: 505-20.

55 Rose F, Benon R. Un cas de presbyophrénie. *L'Encéphale* 1910; **1**: 348-52.

56 Kraepelin E. *Psychiatrie. Ein Lehrbuch für Studierende und Ärzte*. 8th Edition, Vol 2, 1st Part. Leipzig: JA Barth, 1910.

57 Ziehen T. Les démences. In: Marie A (ed). *Traité International de Psychologie Pathologique*. Vol 2. Paris: Alcan, 1911: pp 281-381.

58 Nöuet H. Presbyophrenia of Wernicke and psychopolyneuritis. *Alienist and Neurologist* 1913; **34**: 141-55.

59 Nöuet H. Presbyophrénie de Wernicke et les psychopolynéuritis. *L'Encéphale* 1911; **6**: 141-52.

60 Wollenberg A. Die dementia paralytica. In: Binswanger O, Siemerling E (eds). *Lehrbuch der Psychiatrie*, 4th Edition. Jena: Fischer, 1915: pp 339-406.

61 Bostroem A. Über Presbyophrenie. *Arch Psychiatrie Nerven-krankenheiten* 1933; **99**: 339-54.

62 Lafora GR. Sobre la presbiofrenia sin confabulaciones. *Archivos de Neurobiología* 1935; **15**: 179-211.

63 Burger-Prinz H, Jacob H. Anatomische und klinische Studien zur senilen Demenz. *Zeit gesamte Neurol Psychiatrie* 1938; **161**: 538-43.

64 Bessière R. La presbyophrénie. *L'Encéphale* 1948; **37**: 313-42.

65 Ey H. Les troubles de la mémoire. Étude N° 9. In: *Études Psychiatriques*, Vol 2. Paris: Desclée et Brouwer, 1950.

66 Ey H, Bernard P, Brisset Ch. *Manuel de Psychiatrie*. Paris: Masson et Cie, 1974.

67 Dide M, Gassiot T. Pathogénie de la presbyophrénie. *Rev Neurol* 1912; **23**: 5-7.

68 Morley JB, Cox FN. Cortical blindness with anosognosia, subsequent simultaneous agnosia and persistent gross recent memory defect. *Proc Aust Assoc Neurol* 1974; **11**: 41-7.

69 Swartz BE, Brust JCM. Anton's syndrome accompanying withdrawal hallucinosis in a blind alcoholic. *Neurology* 1984; **34**: 969-73.

70 Traub R, Gajdusek DC, Gibbs CJ. Transmissible virus dementia: The relation of transmissible spongiform encephalopathy to Creutzfeldt-Jakob disease. In: Kinsbourne M, Smith L (eds). *Aging and Dementia*. New York: Spectrum Publications, 1977: pp 91-172.

71 Creutzfeldt HG. Über eine eigenartige herdförmige Erkrankungen des Zentralnervensystem. *Zeit gesamte Neurol Psychiatrie* 1920; **57**: 1-18.

72 Jakob A. Über eine multiplen Sklerose klinisch nahestehende Erkrankung des Zentralnervensystem (spastiche Pseudosklerose) mit bemerkenswertem anatomischem Befunde. Mitteilung eines vierten Falles. *Med Klin* 1921; **17**: 372-6.

73 Richardson EP. Introduction. In: Rottenberg DA, Hochberg FH (eds). *Neurological Classics in Modern Translation*. New York: Hafner Press, 1977: pp 95-6.

74 Gajdusek DC, Zigas V. Degenerative disease of the central nervous system in New Guinea. The endemic occurrence of 'kuru' in the native population. *N Engl J Med* 1957; **257**: 974-8.

75 Hadlow WJ. Scrapie and kuru. *Lancet* 1959; **ii**: 289-90.

76   Gibbs CJ, Gajdusek DC, Asher DM *et al.* Creutzfeldt-Jakob disease: transmission to the chimpanzee. *Science* 1968; **161**: 388-9.

77   Neary D, Snowden JS, Northen B, Goulding P. Dementia of Frontal lobe type. *J Neurol Neurosurg Psychiatry* 1988; **51**: 353-61.

78   Russell JD, Roxanas MG. Psychiatry and the frontal lobes. *Aust NZ J Psychiatry* 1990; **24**: 113-32.

79   Caron M. *Étude clinique de la maladie de Pick.* Paris: Vigot Frères, 1934.

80   Gratiolet LP. *Mémoires sur les plis cérébraux de l'homme et des primates.* Paris: Bertrand, 1854.

81   Anonymous. An exposure of the unphilosophical and unchristian expedients adopted by antiphrenologists, for the purpose of obstructing the moral tendencies of phrenology. A review of John Wayte's book. *The Phrenological Journal and Miscellany* 1832; **7**: 615-22.

82   Broca P. Perte de la parole, ramollissement chronique et destruction partielle du lobe anterieur gauche du cerveau. *Bull Soc Anthrop Paris* 1861; **2**: 235-8.

83   Henderson VH. Paul Broca's less heralded contributions to aphasia research. Historical perspective and contemporary relevance. *Arch Neurol* 1986; **43**: 609-12.

84   Jackson H. The factors of insanities. *Medical Press and Circular* 1894; **ii**: 615-25.

85   Meynert T. *Psychiatry. A clinical treatise on diseases of the fore-brain.* Translated by B Sachs. New York: Putnam, 1885.

86   Pick A. Über die Beziehungen der senilen Hirnatrophie zur Aphasie. *Prager Medicinische Wochenschrift* 1892; **17**: 165-7.

87   Pick A. Senile Hirnatrophie als Grundlage von Herder-scheinungen. *Wiener klinische Wochenschrift* 1901; **14**: 403-4.

88   Pick A. Über einen weiterer Symptomenkomplex im Rahmen der Dementia senilis, bedingt durch umschriebene stärkere Hirnatrophie (gemische Apraxie). *Monatschrift für Psychiatrie und Neurologie* 1906; **19**: 97-108.

89   Barrett AM. Presenile, arteriosclerotic and senile disorders of the brain and cord. In: White WA, Jelliffe SE (eds). *The Modern Treatment of Nervous and Mental Diseases.* London: Kimpton, 1910: pp 675-709.

90   Van Mansvelt J. *Pick's disease.* Enschede: Van der Loeff, 1954.

91   Schneider C. Über Picksche Krankheit. *Monatschrift für Psychiatrie und Neurologie* 1927; **65**: 230-75.

92   Schneider C. Weitere Beiträge zur Lehre von der Pickschen Krankheit. *Zeit gesamte Neurol Psychiatrie* 1929; **120**: 340-84.

93   Marie A. *La démence.* Paris: Doin, 1906.

Chapter 8
Dementia in Shakespeare's King Lear

1   Johnson Samuel. *Plays of William Shakespeare*. London, 1765.
2   Lamb Charles & Mary. *Tales from Shakespeare*. London: Ward Lock, 1807.
3   *Holinshed's Chronicle*. Everyman's Library. London: Dent, 1969.
4   Howells JG. *Family Psychiatry*. Edinburgh: Oliver & Boyd, 1963.
5   Neugebauer R. Medieval & early modern theories of mental illness. *Arch Gen Psych* 1979; **36**: 477-883.
6   Howells JG. *Principles of Family Psychiatry*. London: Pitman, 1976.
7   Howells JG, Osborn ML. The incidence of emotional disorder in a seventeenth-century medical practice. *Med Hist* 1970; **14**: 192-8.
8   Joseph H. *John Hall, Man and Physician*. Hamden, Connecticut: Archon Books, 1964.
9   Bright T. *A Treatise of Melancholie*. London: Vautmollier, 1586.
10 Wilson J Dover. *What Happens in Hamlet*. London: Cambridge University Press, 1964.
11 Esquirol JE. *Mental Maladies, a Treatise on Insanity*. Philadelphia: Lea & Blanchard, 1845.
12 Howells JG, Osborn L. *Abnormal Psychology in Shakespeare's Plays*. Unpublished manuscript.
13 Jackson JH. *Selected Writings*. Taylor J (ed). New York: Basic Books, 1958.
14 Jordan Edward. *A Brief Discourse of a Disease Called The Suffocation of the Mother*. London: Windet, 1603.

Index

Note: page numbers in italic refer to illustrations

List of Contributors

G. C. Berrios Consultant and University Lecturer in Psychiatry, Department of Psychiatry, University of Cambridge; Honorary Librarian, Royal College of Psychiatrists, London, UK

C. H. Cahn Associate Professor of Psychiatry, McGill University, Montreal, Canada

T. Dening Consultant Psychogeriatrician, Fulbourn Hospital, Cambridge, UK

H. L. Freeman Editor, British Journal of Psychiatry; Honorary Professor, University of Salford; Honorary Consultant Psychiatrist, Salford Health Authority, UK

P. Hoff Professor of Psychiatry, Psychiatrische Klinik und Poliklinik, University of Munich, Germany

J. Howells Emeritus Consultant Psychiatrist and former Director, Institute of Family Psychiatry, Ipswich, UK